The Aftermath of Rape

This book documents the journey of the survivors of sexual violence as they navigate the gruelling criminal justice and healthcare systems and the stigma and hostility in their communities in the aftermath of the incident.

Through personal narratives of survivors and their family members, this book examines critical gaps in the existing networks of criminal procedure, health, and rehabilitation for survivors of sexual violence and rape. Using qualitative research, this book distils the narratives gathered through interviews with survivors and their family members to understand their experiences and recommendations. This book contributes to the corpus of literature on different forms of violence against women in India, with an emphasis on understanding the effectiveness of institutions, both formal and informal, in responding to sexual violence and offering suggestions for changes in the health and support systems available to them. It documents post-incident interactions of survivors with family, community, the police, courts, lawyers, and hospitals and highlights the impact of rape on physical and mental health, work, relationships, education, and housing for survivors and their families.

This book will be of interest to those engaged in providing support to survivors of sexual violence, as well as students and researchers of social work and social policy, health and social care, law, gender studies, human rights and civil liberties, gender and sexuality, social welfare, and mental health.

Padma Bhate-Deosthali has extensive experience in research, training, and policy advocacy in the areas of gender-based violence, gender in medical education, health policy research, regulation of the private health sector, and women and work, with a focus on health and human rights. She led CEHAT as its director for eleven years. She was a member of the steering group of the GDG-WHO for developing policy and clinical practice guidelines for responding to violence against women and also a member of the National

Committee under the MoHFW for drafting the "Guidelines and protocols for medico-legal care for victims/survivors of sexual violence" in 2014. She coordinated the setting up of Dilaasa, a public hospital-based crisis centre on domestic violence in Mumbai.

Sangeeta Rege has a master's degree in social work. She has eighteen years of experience in engaging the public health sector on gender-based violence and, more recently, on integrating gender concerns in medical education. She is presently the coordinator of the CEHAT. Sangeeta is trained in social science research, advocacy, training, and counselling and has led CEHAT's legal interventions to facilitate gender-sensitive medico-legal care for survivors of sexual violence from 2010. She has led the upscaling of the Dilaasa hospital-based crisis centres in different states of India and is committed to generating evidence to strengthen the role of health systems in responding to VAW. She has co-edited a book for Routledge titled *Violence against Women and Girls: Understanding Responses and Approaches in the Indian Health Sector* (2020).

Sanjida Arora has been associated with CEHAT for the past seven years. She is a trained dentist and holds a degree of master in public health from Tata Institute of Social Science. She co-led an implementation research project in collaboration with the WHO to test training approaches for the rollout of the WHO Clinical and Policy Guidelines, 2013, in two medical colleges of Maharashtra. She was also the principal investigator on a research project on assessing the effectiveness of counselling intervention in antenatal departments of public hospitals for women facing domestic violence. She has been leading the capacity building of several civil society organizations in data management and analysis of counselling service records in a rigorous and ethical manner that protects the confidentiality and anonymity of survivors.

The Aftermath of Rape

Survivors Speak

**Padma Bhate-Deosthali,
Sangeeta Rege and Sanjida Arora**

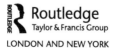

Routledge
Taylor & Francis Group

LONDON AND NEW YORK

First published 2022
by Routledge
4 Park Square, Milton Park, Abingdon, Oxon OX14 4RN

and by Routledge
605 Third Avenue, New York, NY 10158

Routledge is an imprint of the Taylor & Francis Group, an informa business

© 2022 Padma Bhate-Deosthali, Sangeeta Rege and Sanjida Arora

British Library Cataloguing-in-Publication Data
A catalogue record for this book is available from the British Library

Library of Congress Cataloging-in-Publication Data
A catalog record for this book has been requested

ISBN: 978-1-032-15145-8 (hbk)
ISBN: 978-1-032-25165-3 (pbk)
ISBN: 978-1-003-28188-7 (ebk)

DOI: 10.4324/9781003281887

Typeset in Times New Roman
by Apex CoVantage, LLC

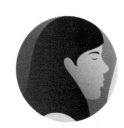
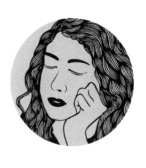
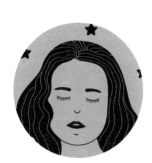
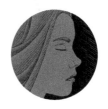
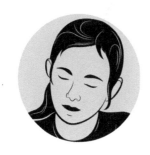

SURVIVING
SEXUAL
VIOLENCE

Designed by Poornima Burte

Contents

Acknowledgements

We are indebted to the survivors for trusting us and making time to share their experiences. Their resolve and resilience were inspiring for us as researchers. We were overwhelmed with the efforts they took to organise their thoughts, the paperwork, and also their reflections and insights into what needed to change to make the aftermath of rape less arduous. Many of them said that their stories must be told to as many people so that others can learn from it.

This is our effort to present their narratives, and we hope that all those involved in responding to sexual violence will benefit from reading them. Their stories have prompted us to improve our interventions with survivors and make them more meaningful and relevant to their lives.

We sincerely acknowledge the contributions of all the researchers and the interventionists who contributed to this project at various stages: Aarthi Chandrasekhar, Amruta Bavadekar, Chitra Joshi, Prachi Avalaskar, Rajeeta Chavan, and Sujata Ayarkar.

We thank the members of the AnusnadhanTrust's Institutional Ethics Committee and Programme Development Committee of CEHAT (Centre for Enquiry into Health and Allied Themes) who ensured the scientific rigour and ethical practice for conducting this research. The report of the study is available on the CEHAT website.

We thank the Azim Premji Philanthropic Initiative for financial support for this research.

Introduction

The public protests following the gang rape of a young health professional in Delhi in December 2012 compelled the Government of India to take cognisance of sexual violence. The government appointed a three-member committee headed by Justice Verma to examine the lacunae in criminal laws and their enforcement in cases of sexual assault against women. Within a month, in January 2013, the Justice Verma Committee (JVC) produced a comprehensive report with a detailed analysis and recommendations. The JVC report mapped the socio-economic, cultural, political, and juridical basis for sexual violence against women. It asserted that rape was a violation of a woman's sexual autonomy and bodily integrity. It noted the hostility, insensitivity, and institutionalised bias against the survivor prevalent in the system across the police, healthcare, and the courts and made incisive recommendations for overhauling these institutions through legislative interventions setting standard gender sensitivity procedures and protocols (Verma et al., 2013).

This was followed by critical changes to the rape law in the country through the Criminal Law (Amendment) Act (CLA) 2013, which expanded the definition of rape to include all forms of sexual violence: penetrative acts (oral, anal, vaginal), including the use of objects/weapons/fingers, and non-penetrative acts (touching, fondling, stalking, disrobing, etc.) It defined consent and clearly stated that lack of resistance (absence of injuries) does not mean consent. (Bhate-Deosthali and Rege, 2015; Government of India [GOI], 2013). The law retains the exception of marital rape from the offence of rape. The concession made by CLA 2013 was to extend the purview of rape to any wife living separately, though entailing a lighter prison sentence. CLA 2013 expanded the categories of aggravated rape beyond the precincts of the police station, jail, hospital, remand home, and women's institution, to include rape in areas under the operation of armed forces; rape by a person in a position of trust, authority, control, or dominance; or rape during communal or sectarian violence. CLA 2013 did not classify caste as a specific category, even though impunity for sexual assault of Dalit women is

DOI: 10.4324/9781003281887-1

endemic (Dubey, 2015). Evidence suggests that transgender persons and men are often subjected to heinous sexual abuse and assault, particularly in police stations and jails and during caste atrocities, necessitating the introduction of specific crimes of sexual assault for their protection, but these need to be pursued (Butalia, 2015).

The law brought in crucial procedural changes and new remedies to make the system responsive to enable survivors to access legal redress. There have been recommendations for restorative justice to victims through state compensation schemes, medico-legal guidelines by the Ministry of Health and Family Welfare (MoHFW), and standard operating procedures (SOPs) for the police (Partners for Law in Development [PLD], 2017). The State of Delhi pioneered in setting up child-friendly courts that issued guidelines for creating an enabling environment in the courts for child survivors. These were positive steps towards reducing the hostility of various institutions, such as the police, hospitals, and courts, towards rape survivors and their families. The law also has provisions for punishing the police and doctors in case they fail to register an FIR (first information report) or provide treatment, respectively. No case has been registered so far for denial of treatment (MoHFW, 2014).

Role of health systems

The protests and campaigns raised several issues connected with justice for rape survivors, and groups such as CEHAT (Centre for Enquiry into Health and Allied Themes) drew attention to the insensitive practices in the health sector. They especially pointed to the use of unscientific and anti-women practices within forensic medicine, such as the use of the two-finger test, which was used wrongly to determine the status of virginity of the survivor and to assess her past sexual history. Several lawyers and activists spoke out against the insensitivity of the health providers. A petition by CEHAT and Human Rights Watch (HRW) against the use of the two-finger test was endorsed by several institutions, researchers, lawyers, and doctors and submitted to the PMO (Human Rights Watch [HRW], 2012; CEHAT, 2012).

The JVC report included an entire chapter that addressed institutional bias to rape within the health system. Amongst the recommendations pertaining to the health sector, one was for developing uniform protocols and guidelines in responding to sexual violence. This included strong recommendations for the removal of insensitive and unscientific procedures that traumatise survivors. The report further recommended the setting up of services for the provision of psychosocial care and rehabilitation of survivors of sexual violence, thus clearly spelling out a major responsibility for the health system in India (Verma et al., 2013).

The CLA 2013 recognised the right to treatment for all survivors of sexual violence in all public and private healthcare facilities. Failure to treat is now an offence under the law. The law further disallows any reference to past sexual practices of the survivor. The CLA 2013 has made a strong case for positively transforming the response of the health sector to sexual violence (GOI, 2013).

Taking cognisance of the lack of uniform protocols and gaps in provision of medico-legal care to survivors of sexual violence, the recommendations of the JVC, the CLA 2013, and Protection of Children from Sexual Offences (POCSO) 2012, the Ministry of Health and Family Welfare (MoHFW) issued the first national directive to the health sector on responding to sexual violence. The Ministry of Health in India included a response to gender-based violence in its policy in 2017 by clearly mandating gender training of health providers, making hospitals women-friendly and providing care to survivors/victims of gender-based violence (National Health Policy, 2017).

Medico-legal guidelines for responding to sexual violence

The health ministry's guidelines provide a clear directive to all health facilities to ensure that survivors of all forms of sexual violence, rape, and incest – including people who face marginalisation based on disability, sexual orientation, caste, religion, and class – have immediate access to healthcare services. They recognise the need to create an enabling environment for survivors to speak out about abuse without fear of being blamed, where they can receive empathetic support in their quest for justice and rebuild their lives after the assault. The protocol requires doctors to seek informed consent or refusal after demystifying the medico-legal procedures and focuses on history and relevant evidence collection. It includes immediate and follow-up treatment, post-rape care (including emergency contraception, post-exposure prophylaxis for HIV prevention, and access to safe abortion services), police protection, emergency shelter, documentation of cases, forensic services and referrals for legal aid, and other services.

The comprehensive gender-sensitive model in Mumbai hospitals

As a strategy, CEHAT focuses on good practice as it has set up a model in collaboration with the MCGM that adheres to international standards of gender sensitivity and is evidence-based. This has been functional in three hospitals since 2008 and has provided comprehensive care and treatment to a large number of rape survivors (Rege et al., 2014). The CEHAT-MCGM initiative provides comprehensive care to all survivors of sexual violence. The model was built on the experience of running two crisis centres for survivors of domestic violence for more than a decade. The core components of this model, which has been functioning in three municipal hospitals since 2008, are as follows:

- Seeking informed consent for all aspects of the medico-legal examination
- Eliciting history of sexual violence and documenting it
- Examination and relevant evidence collection
- Formulating a medical opinion based on history, clinical findings, and forensic evidence
- Providing treatment and psychosocial support
- Maintaining a chain of custody

The focus has been on informed consent, detailed documentation of the assault, formulation of medical opinion based on clinical findings, factors leading to the possible loss of evidence (such as reporting delay and bathing/douching/menstruating/urinating), circumstances of abuse (such as verbal threats and numbing due to fear), and so on.

An important component of the CEHAT-MCGM model is building the capacity of healthcare providers to carry out medico-legal examinations, understand the impact and health consequences of assault, and the provision of care. The training also includes a perspective on the dynamics of sexual violence and the myths related to it to enable them to overcome biases. A crisis interventionist is available at all times, responding to any query of the examining physicians, dealing with the police and the Child Welfare Committee (CWC), and providing crisis intervention services to the survivor and her family. The work being carried out by CEHAT and the MCGM to provide comprehensive care to all survivors of sexual violence is significant in this context as it provides a pathway for what the MoHFW needs to do in terms of setting up and monitoring of services through rigorous training, hand-holding, and analysing the service records. The study on the aftermath of rape is to understand the experiences of survivors after they leave the hospital where a sensitive and standard care is provided to them.

The hospitals have been able to harness all available technical support, such as lawyers, social workers, translators, and special educators, amongst others, and have been able to interface with the police, the CWC, and courts effectively. The hospitals have thus been able to address the needs of boys, transgender persons, and persons with disabilities, in addition to girls and women. As a regular practice, trained doctors seek to establish a rapport with the survivor directly and enable her to speak out without getting carried away or limiting themselves to the history given to police. This is an important aspect that must become routine practice in all health facilities. Often the police and parents bring girls who may have run away from home or "gone missing" and expect doctors to rule out rape, or in the case of women, the police and family want to know if she was raped. The expectation here is for doctors to check if there are injuries and/or if the hymen is intact. Neither of these is present in many cases of rape.

Survivors coming forward

The campaign following the Nirbhaya incident and legal amendments created a lot of awareness about rape, as evidenced in a rise in reporting of all cases of sexual violence but more amongst adolescents and adult women. According to the National Crime Records Bureau (NCRB), an office located in the Ministry of Home Affairs, after the changes initiated in the law, there was a 56.3% increase in the number of criminal complaints reported to the police in 2016 (38,9,47) compared to 2012 (24,923). The sustained campaign and the changes in the law have had an impact on society in general and on the reporting of sexual violence.

Table 0.1 Reported cases of sexual violence (SV)

	2012	2013	2014	2015	2016
Rape	24,923	33,707	3,6735	3,4651	38,947
Other forms of SV	54,524	83,328	9,6202	9,5541	90,375

Source: NCRB (2012, 2013, 2014, 2015, 2016) https://ncrb.gov.in/en

Recent evidence based on the NCRB data found that fewer than 1.5% of the victims of sexual violence in India report their assaults to the police, though there is some indication of increased reporting of incidents of rape to the police following a very high-profile fatal gang rape in Delhi in December 2012. A similar observation has been made in a CEHAT study based on hospital records that found that the numbers had increased threefold post the incident in Mumbai. However, the conviction rates remain as low as 18% (NCRB, 2016).

Rationale for the study

There are no studies on the impact of sexual violence on survivors in India. To the best of our knowledge, we have not come across studies following the life experiences of survivors of rape. It is essential to document the life experiences of survivors post-rape as this would help in understanding the impact of the incident on their health, relationships, and work and the challenges faced by them after reporting rape to the police or hospital. This research is a first that brings to the fore the voices of survivors and their families that could transform the current response to sexual violence.

Sources of data

The primary sources of data for the study are in-depth interviews with adult survivors and parents of child and adolescent survivors. Between April 2008 and March 2015, there were 728 survivors who came to three hospitals for their medico-legal examination (CEHAT, 2018). All of them were approached, and after discussing their current status, which included their health and safety and the status of their case, amongst other things, the interventionist informed them about the purpose of the study and sought their oral consent for participation. They were informed that their participation in the study was completely voluntary and their refusal would have no effect on the services being provided to them. Before the interview, the researcher read the service records to understand the entire history and background. This ensured that the respondent did not have to repeat any information that was already available. In the case of survivors younger than 18, the parent was interviewed.

Objectives of the study

1   To understand the experiences of the survivor/family and document their interface with informal systems, such as family (immediate and extended) and community, and formal systems, such as the police, courts, lawyers, and hospitals
2   To enquire into the impact of rape on their physical and mental health, work, relationships, education, and housing/shelter (Impact is defined as consequences on physical health, mental health, employment, education, income, and interface with the community.)

Data collection

The data collection for the study was initiated at the end of December 2016, and the last interview was conducted in February 2018. The interventionists approached the survivors by either calling them on their safe telephone numbers and/or by sending letters to the address intimated by them. Of all the survivors, 87% (634) could be contacted either by phone or by letter or both. Telephone numbers were available for 63% of the survivors, that is, 457 of the 728 survivors. Of these, in 170 cases, the numbers were not available or out of service or did not exist or were not in use. Potential survivors who could be contacted over the phone numbered 287 (63%). The addresses of 578 survivors (79%) were available.

The team was able to establish contact with only 25% (181) of the survivors. Of those that could be contacted, 36% (66) participated in the study, 23% refused to participate, 7% agreed but did not turn up for the interview, 28% were reluctant to speak and expressed concern as the case was ongoing, 2% expressed the need for intervention, and 4% had relocated and so could not come for the interview.

Of the 66 research participants, 5 required intervention based on the initial contact made by the interventionist, and so it was provided before the interview. Nearly 25 of the research participants did not express any need for intervention at the time of contact, but participation in the interview process helped them to identify intervention needs. All of them were provided with various support services after the interview. The interviews were conducted at the place of the survivor's choice. Most of them were conducted at the CEHAT office or in one of the *Dilaasa* centres. Two were held in the offices of the respondent, one at home and one outside a church. The interviews were conducted by a team comprising a researcher and an interventionist to enable immediate psychological support during or after the interview.

Ethical considerations

The team recognises the specific vulnerabilities of survivors of violence, and therefore, the first call made to each of them was by an interventionist (trained counsellor) to enquire about the well-being of the survivor, her family, her education, her health, and her interface with the hospital, police, and court and offer any type of intervention required. If an intervention was required, that was offered first. Only after this was the study introduced and consent sought for participation. It is important to state here that the consent was sought over multiple calls across a few weeks, which allowed the family to make the decision about participation. The fact that 23% refused to participate and 28% expressed that they were reluctant to participate in the study indicates that this process was followed strictly and those who consented to participate did so freely without any inhibitions.

The consent form was read out slowly and clearly at the time of the interview in the language that the survivors were comfortable in. The consent forms were available in English, Hindi, and Marathi. All aspects of the study were explained. Six research participants refused to have their interviews recorded, and their decision was respected. In one of these cases, the father refused to sign the consent letter, saying that their lawyer had told them not to sign any paper. Therefore, in this case, only oral consent was sought. The names of all the interviewees were also changed to protect their anonymity.

Reimbursement and compensation

It was decided that a token amount of INR 400 would be given to each research participant to compensate for the travel expenses and loss of wages. At the end of the interview, when the token amount was given, all the respondents refused to accept the money. They expressed their gratitude for the work being done by the team and said that they felt good after talking to them. Hence, they did not want to take any money. It had to be explained to them that an ethics committee that reviews the work of the team had decided on the compensation, and they were persuaded to accept the amount.

Summarising the results

The experiences of the research participants in a study conducted by CEHAT to understand the impact of sexual violence tells us that surviving sexual violence is tough and the entire family suffers at various levels. Survivors continue to be turned away, be blamed, be denied treatment, face hostility at all levels, and be stuck in long legal procedures. Using a qualitative research design, the study "Surviving Sexual Violence: Impact of Survivors and Families" (Bhate-Deosthali et al., 2018) applied the ecological framework to interview survivors and/or their family members to understand the experience of disclosing incident/s of sexual violence and their experience thereafter with the hospital and document their interface with informal systems, such as family (immediate and extended) and community, and formal systems, such as the police, courts, lawyers, and hospitals. It also enquired into the impact of rape on their physical and mental health, work, relationships, education, and housing/shelter. The impact was defined as consequences on physical health, mental health, employment, education, income, and interface with the community. Of the 66 respondents, only 2 had decided not to enter the CJS (criminal justice system). Few decided not to proceed with the case after it came up for hearing. But the rest of them had gone through the entire process or were in the process when they were interviewed.

What emerges is the impact of secondary victimisation that survivors and their families have to suffer. Institutional practices and values that place the needs of the organisation above the needs of clients or patients are implicated in the problem. Even very basic expectations from the police, such as registering the complaint immediately, being treated with dignity, and being taken seriously when they report continued threats and violence by the perpetrator, were not met. Calling them repeatedly to the police station and asking them to repeat what happened was a common experience too. The health system also did not create a conducive environment for all survivors. While immediate treatment was provided, the long-term health consequences remain unaddressed. The court experience was overwhelming for most as they were left to themselves to deal with the CJS and its procedural rigmarole.

It is known that survivors who come out and report rape are fewer than the ones who do not speak out due to "family honour". Rape is seen as a loss of honour and not as violence inflicted on women. "A woman lost her chastity/modesty/honour" and "Rape is worse than death" are notions that are deeply patriarchal. The cliché of rape as a "fate worse than death" for women valorises virginity even as it simultaneously reduces her worth – or lack of it – to the condition of the hymen and goes hand in hand with another trope: that the women who get raped are women who ask for it. These notions focus on individual women and do not recognise the use of sexual violence as a systematic tool to oppress and silence women. These notions also create stereotypes of good and bad victims. A woman's character, her past relationships, whether she reported rape immediately or after, whether she had any marks of injury on her (did she struggle enough?), and many such biases and prejudices are deeply entrenched in the way society and institutions respond to her. As a result, not only is the rape survivor rendered worthless, but this internally conflicted victim-temptress combination recoils on the survivor, depriving her of both value and voice and freeing perpetrators from the responsibility for the crime. (Butalia and Murthy, 2018)

Rapists are created by a society that devalues women and promotes rape culture. Cross-cultural studies have found reliable differences between "rape-prone" and "rape-free" societies. In her study of 156 tribal societies, Sanday (1981) found "rape-prone" societies were more gender inequitable and aggressive. The genders were more segregated, women were less powerful, ideas of male dominance prevailed, and war and interpersonal violence were common.

It is evidenced that the journey of survivors who gather the courage to disclose is not easy as they face unsupportive reactions from individuals and institutions (Ullman, 2000). The wide acceptance of rape myths make rape a peculiar offence where victim blaming is more common than any other crime (Grubb and Harrower, 2008; Bieneck and Krahé, 2011). Victim blaming has been associated with increased feelings of guilty suicidal ideation, shame, low self-esteem and self-blame amongst survivors (Kubany et al., 1995; Ullman et al., 2007). The personal beliefs and behaviours of social service workers are also sources of secondary victimisation.

The sociocultural level concerns the macrosystem that provides the "cultural scaffolding" (Gavey and Schmidt, 2011, as cited in Sonpar, 2018) that supports sexual violence. It refers to the norms, practices and discourses of sex, gender, and violence prevailing in a society that set up the preconditions for sexual violence to occur. It includes the construction of rape myths that circulate in a culture. There are socially learned, stereotyped beliefs about rape, rape victims, and rapists (Burt, 1998) that justify sexual violence against women and advocate that women are responsible for their sexual victimisation. Despite their falsehood, they are endorsed by a substantial segment of the population and permeate legal, media, and religious institutions (Edwards et al., 2011).

Some examples are as follows: forced sex between intimate partners is not really rape, women secretly want to be forced and can prevent it if they really want, and women who get raped somehow deserve it (because they are promiscuous or engage in unfeminine behaviour, such as being sexually assertive or going to bars alone). Beliefs about male sexuality also contribute to a distorted understanding of rape, specifically the idea that men cannot control their sexual urges. There are also myths about what constitute "real rape". An examination of a large number of victim narratives found that one in five women who disclosed an incident of sexual violence excused or justified it, largely drawing on stereotypes that male sexual aggression is natural and normal within dating relationships or is the victim's fault (Weiss, 2009).

These can manifest as belief in rape myths that blame the victim for the assault and which result in providers voicing doubt about the veracity of the victims' accounts, neglecting to offer important services such as pregnancy testing, informing rape survivors about HIV/AIDS and other sexually transmitted diseases, and legal prosecution of the sexual assault and the performance of services in ways that leave victims feeling "violated and re-raped" or which otherwise damage the victims' psychological well-being.

Survivors spoke about victim blaming and entrenched manifestations of rape myths in the way they described the unsupportive neighbourhood and the unsupportive responses from the public institutions that they had approached for redress and justice.

This re-traumatisation burdens the survivor and her family, increases stress, and prevents recovery from rape, as evidenced in the ongoing trauma and health consequences that the survivor and/or her family members are still suffering even four to seven years after the incident. The respondents strongly recommended the need for a support person to handhold, explain the various steps in the CJS, and help them navigate the system.

Applying the ecological model to the experiences of respondents, we present the aftermath of reporting rape at different levels:

The study found that at the individual level, factors such as nature of assault, age, and other sociodemographic variables did not have a direct bearing on health consequences and well-being. All of them reported immediate and/or long-term health consequences. Survivors of all ages came forward and disclosed various forms of sexual violence, such as touching, attempt to rape, and penetrative assaults.

The relationship with the abuser had a bearing on the mental health of the survivor. In cases where the abuser was an intimate partner, survivors suffered a psychological impact, including suicidal ideation and attempts at suicide. For those who were sexually abused by intimate partners, the feeling of betrayal and being cheated was deep – and so was the feeling that the perpetrator must be punished. Similarly, those survivors and their family members who had to live with continued threats from the abuser and/or his family reported high stress levels and living in constant fear and anxiety. The sexual nature of the assault was a major barrier in accessing healthcare, especially reproductive health services, and it also caused acute anxiety amongst young girls about whether the future partner would come to know about the incident, whether she would be able to bear a child and so on. We did not speak directly to children, but parents spoke about how they had helped them cope with it.

At the micro level, the study looked at the response of the immediate and extended family members. It was found that the family was supportive of children and adolescents. They tried to create a safe and healing environment for the children but restricted their mobility in many ways. The notions that "good girls" do not spend a lot of time outside the house and pubertal girls must wear layered clothing[1] were reported by some.

For those who had eloped or had been cheated by their partners (sexual intercourse on the false promise to marry) or raped by their husbands, the family was not supportive. They blamed the survivor for what had happened. These survivors found themselves lonely and under immense pressure due to the attitude of the family as there was a constant feeling that they had brought disgrace to the entire family.

The notion that punishing the accused is the only way that society will believe that the survivor is telling the truth is deep-rooted to such an extent that the families dread a negative court outcome. This is stronger amongst adult women and adolescent girls due to the victim blaming that they had to encounter. A young woman burnt herself, and her brother perceived this as the only option and right step taken by her, which ensured justice for her.

At the meso level, the study looked at the response of the police, hospitals, and courts. It was found that all three institutions were hostile and tough to navigate. The rape survivor was doubted and seen with suspicion from the police station to the court. Registering an FIR, which is the first step towards accessing justice, was an arduous process. The negative experiences in these institutions had a long-lasting impact on the survivors and their families.

They had to face victim blaming at all institutions, and it was disturbing that very few had positive experiences with the police and courts. The only exception was hospitals, where most did not report negative experiences, which can be attributed to the presence of a crisis intervention department in these hospitals that brought them in touch with a counsellor/social worker who helped them navigate the system. Similarly, a few had support from NGOs, which was crucial in mitigating problems with the police and/or accessing other services. The experience of the young girls who were forced to run away with their boyfriends due to domestic violence from their natal families highlights the ordeal of what the couple has to go through because of the criminalisation of consensual sex amongst adolescents. This requires urgent amendment in the law.

At the macro level, the study explored the interaction with the larger community, neighbourhood, workplace, and schools in which survivors live and operate. It was found that the broader social environment was wrought with rape myths and a predominant rape culture. Nearly 20% of the survivors had to relocate to another place due to the victim-blaming attitude of the community, which calls for changing the mindset. Overall, the ecosystem is that of disbelief of all rape survivors. The families found themselves completely isolated as most people around them did not want to associate with a family that had filed a rape case. There was a lot of pressure, both direct and indirect, to settle the matter as the abuser was mostly from the same area. Parents were instructed by school authorities to change school or not send the child till the case was over. The lack of faith in the school system is evidenced by the fact that families of only 5 of the 45 child and adolescent informed the school about what had happened. Many employers asked the survivor's parents to leave the job as they feared that the police would come to the workplace repeatedly. All these interactions stigmatised the survivors and their families, impacted their social interaction, and deeply affected their economic well-being. The perceptions that granting of bail and acquittal meant that the girl/woman was lying or that it was a false case were so strong that these led to taunts and harassment of the survivors and their families, causing them agony and making them feel helpless.

At the chrono system, the study explored the impact of other forms of discrimination. The study found that some of the survivors had to face multiple traumas, such as abuse from more than one person, continued abuse, and threats from the abuser, which had a debilitating effect on them. These were survivors who also experienced severe violations at the level of the police station and courts, which compounded the matter and made it more difficult for them to carry on their daily tasks and live with dignity. Class, gender, caste, and community deeply impact the reporting and the consequences of reporting. The responses of the formal and informal systems to survivors and their families explored in this study are enmeshed in the way the abuse and the class, caste, and community of the survivors interplay. It does not impact all survivors in the same way.

Note

1 Young girls are often asked to wear several layers of clothing to hide the pubertal changes in the body to avoid male gaze.

References

Bhate-Deosthali, P., and Rege, S. (2015). Implications of the changes in rape law on health sector. In M. Verwoerd and C. Lopes (Eds.), *A case for paradigm shift in sexualised violence in the national debate cross border observations on India and South Africa* (pp. 130–139). Heinrich Böll Foundation Southern Africa.

Bhate-Deosthali, P., Rege, S., Arora, S., Avlaskar, P., Chavan, R., and Bavadekar, A. (2018). *Surviving sexual violence: Impact on survivors and families.* Centre for Enquiry into Health and Allied Themes.

Bieneck, S., and Krahé, B. (2011). Blaming the victim and exonerating the perpetrator in cases of rape and robbery: Is there a double standard? *Journal of Interpersonal Violence, 26*(9), 1785–1797. https://doi.org/10.1177/0886260510372945

Burt, M. R. (1998). Rape myths. In M. E. Odem and J. Clay-Warner (Eds.), *Confronting rape and sexual assault* (pp. 129–144). Scholarly Resources.

Butalia, U. (2015). December 16th 2012: A rape, a murder and a movement. In M. Verwoerd and C. Lopes (Eds.), *A case for paradigm shift in sexualised violence in the national debate cross border observations on India and South Africa* (pp. 78–97). Heinrich Böll Foundation Southern Africa.

Butalia, U., and Murthy, L. (Eds.). (2018). *Breaching the citadel: The India papers I.* Zubaan.

Centre for Enquiry into Health and Allied Themes (CEHAT). (2012). *Establishing a comprehensive health sector response to sexual assault.* Centre for Enquiry into Health and Allied Themes.

Centre for Enquiry into Health and Allied Themes (CEHAT). (2018). *Understanding dynamics of sexual violence: a study of case records.* Centre for Enquiry into Health and Allied Themes.

Contractor, S., Divekar, R., and Rajan, A (CEHAT). (2000). *Report on observations conducted at the police hospital.* Centre for Enquiry into Health and Allied Themes.

Dubey, P. (2015, July 11). A portrait of the Indian as a young dalit girl [blog post]. *Twocircles.net.* http://twocircles.net/2015jul11/1436593643.html; http://in.news.yahoo.com/a-portrait-of-the-indian-as-a-young-dalit-girl-034726310.html

Edwards, K. M., Turchik, J. A., Dardis, C. M., Reynolds, N., and Gidycz, C. A. (2011). Rape myths: History, individual and institutional-level presence, and implications for change. *Sex Roles, 65,* 761–773. https://doi.org/10.1007% 2Fs11199-011-9943-2

Gavey, N., and Schmidt, J. (2011). "Trauma of rape" discourse: A double-edged template for everyday understandings of the impact of rape? *Violence Against Women, 17*(4), 433–456. https://doi.org/10.1177/1077801211404194

Government of India. (2013). *Criminal law (amendment) act (2013).* Government of India.

Grubb, A., and Harrower, J. (2008). Attribution of blame in cases of rape: An analysis of participant gender, type of rape and perceived similarity to the victim. *Aggression and Violent Behavior, 13*(5), 396–405. https://doi.org/10.1016/j. avb.2008.06.006

Human Rights Watch. (2012). *India: Joint letter to prime minister Dr. Manmohan Singh: Ensure police are held accountable for gender-based violence.* www.hrw. org/news/2012/05/14/india-joint-letter-prime-minister-dr-manmohan-singh

Ministry of Health and Family Welfare. (2014). *Guidelines and protocols: Medico-legal care for survivors/victims of sexual violence.* Government of India.

Ministry of Women and Child Development. (2012). *The protection of children from sexual offences act (2012).* Government of India.

National Crime Records Bureau (NCRB). (2012). *Crime in India 2012.* Ministry of Home Affairs, Government of India. https://ncrb.gov.in/en/crime-india-year-2012

National Crime Records Bureau (NCRB). (2013). *Crime in India 2013.* Ministry of Home Affairs, Government of India. https://ncrb.gov.in/en/crime-india-year-2013

National Crime Records Bureau (NCRB). (2014). *Crime in India 2014.* Ministry of Home Affairs, Government of India. https://ncrb.gov.in/en/crime-india-year-2014

National Crime Records Bureau (NCRB). (2015). *Crime in India 2015: Statistics.* Ministry of Home Affairs, Government of India. https://ncrb.gov.in/en/crime-india-year-2015

National Crime Records Bureau (NCRB). (2016). *Crime in India 2016: Statistics.* Ministry of Home Affairs, Government of India. https://ncrb.gov.in/en/crime-india-2016-0

National Health Policy. (2017). Ministry of Health and Family Welfare. https://main.mohfw.gov.in/sites/default/files/9147562941489753121.pdf

Partners for Law in Development. (2017). *Towards victim friendly responses and procedures for prosecuting rape: A study of pre-trial and trial stages of rape prosecutions in Delhi (January 2014–March 15).*

Rege, S., Bhate-Deosthali, P., Reddy, J. N., and Contractor, S. (2014). Responding to sexual violence: Evidence-based model for the health sector. *Economic and Political Weekly, 49*(48), 96–101.

Sanday, P. R. (1981). The socio-cultural context of rape: A cross-cultural study. *Journal of Social Issues, 37*(4), 5–27. https://doi.org/10.1111/j.1540-4560.1981. tb01068.x

Sonpar, S. (2018). Sexual violence and impunity: A psychosocial perspective. In U. Butalia and L. Murthy (Eds.), *Breaching the citadel: The India papers I* (pp. 235–293). Zubaan.

Ullman, S. E. (2000). Psychometric characteristics of the social reactions questionnaire: A measure of reactions to sexual assault victims. *Psychology of Women Quarterly, 24*(3), 257–271. https://doi.org/10.1111/j.1471-6402.2000.tb00208.x

Ullman, S. E., Townsend, S. M., Filipas, H. H., and Starzynski, L. L. (2007). Structural models of the relations of assault severity, social support, avoidance coping, self-blame, and PTSD among sexual assault survivors. *Psychology of Women Quarterly, 31*(1), 23–37. https://doi.org/10.1111/j.1471-6402.2007.00328.x

Verma, J. S., Seth, L., Subramanian, G., and Justice JS Verma Committee. (2013). *Report of the committee on amendments to criminal law*. Government of India.

Weiss, K. G. (2009). "Boys will be boys" and other gendered accounts: An exploration of victims' excuses and justification for unwanted sexual contact and coercion. *Violence Against Women, 15*(7), 810–834. https://doi.org/10.1177/1077801209333611

1 Contextualising the survivors' narratives

The seven narratives of survivors bring to fore their journey from the incident of violence to navigating various systems and the effect it had on them and their family members. The research participants had all come for the interview well prepared with all their papers. They said that they would like others to learn from their experience so that there is a change and other survivors don't suffer as they did. Each one of them said that they felt better after talking about their experiences. They expressed a feeling of hope, relief, satisfaction, unburdening of all their angst. Most of them, including their fathers, cried in the interview and said that participation in the study was cathartic.

The seven narratives have been selected to highlight the multitude of ways in which survivors and their families are affected after they report a case of sexual violence. They are of varying ages who suffered different forms of sexual violence: Two children aged 4 years and 6 years were sexually abuse, three young girls aged 15–16 years were kidnapped, brutally assaulted, and raped. One girl suffered a disability. An adult woman was raped by a person known in the community. Finally, a married woman recorded a case of marital rape. Vulnerabilities based on disability, economic status, and community make the entire journey arduous. The formal processes are bereft of any sensitivity to the circumstances of the survivors but have to be followed to get justice. The institutionalised biases across various systems and the rape culture so ingrained affect the survivor and her family in myriad ways. The role of the community in further isolating them and, in turn, blaming the survivor for what happened to her has a deep impact. In the absence of well-designed and relevant support services, the survivors and their families have built their resilience to cope with the situation.

These narratives bring in the impact of this hostility of formal institutions and that of ostracisation by neighbourhood and community on the survivors. The consequences on a survivor are based on socio-economic conditions, politics, and geographic location. The journey of a survivor is

DOI: 10.4324/9781003281887-2

determined by the location of the perpetrator and the context in which violence is inflicted – there are multiple vulnerabilities that a survivor and her family have to endure. The road to justice is as complex and gruelling as daily living and survival. The focus on the CJS is on conviction/acquittal and does nothing to aid the rebuilding of her life. Access to education and livelihood and a change in social attitudes need as much attention.

This re-traumatisation adds to the trauma of the survivor and her family, increases stress, and prevents recovery from rape as evidenced in the ongoing trauma and health consequences that the survivor and/or her family members are still suffering even four to seven years after the incident. As evidenced in other studies, the respondents strongly recommended the need for a support person to handhold, explain the various steps in the CJS, and help them navigate the system.

Ria's mother narrated the incident and all that had happened as though it happened just yesterday. Ria was 4 years old when she was raped by a young boy close to their family. Even nine years after the incident, she said, "No mother can ever forget such an incident." She spoke about the insensitivity of the police and how a WPC "checked" the genitals of her daughter at the police station. The incident caused her a lot of pain and hurt as the abuser and his family were neighbours and close family friends. He was like a son to her. They had to deal with a lot of pressure to not register the case, but they were determined. However, the system broke them, and they informed the court that they didn't want to pursue it due to the delay in court hearings. She felt that her daughter would never be able to move ahead if this went on for so many years. Despite their determination and willingness to bear the social and economic cost of travelling to court, they decided to stop going to court. Her daughter is now smart and bold, and she had taken care to not mar her daughter's future with this incident. She and her family were isolated in their community as people distanced themselves, and reference to the incident came up repeatedly. They have been accused of making a false case and ridiculed for having withdrawn the case.

Sara's story of fortitude involves a father who has decided not to give in to the threats and abuse from the abuser and his politically connected family. This is a migrant family from Uttar Pradesh, and the abuser belongs to a family that is actively involved with a local political party. He had to quit a regular salaried job and work irregular and long hours with less pay. But he has done it as he has resolved to not withdraw the case. As he said, "I have told them you can come and kill me, no problem." Being a Muslim man married to a Hindu woman, the family has been experiencing threats and social isolation for years. In all this hostile environment, he has nurtured his daughter and helped her cope with what happened, and made her fearless.

Bindu is now married and doing well, but her mother spoke of the trauma that Bindu had to suffer when she was kidnapped and raped by a boy living in their neighbourhood. Bindu suffered severe genital injuries and infections that took months to heal. The family endured all the hostility and threats and persuasion from the local leaders who were close to the abuser's family with the hope to get justice. They were also disappointed as the court opined that the girl had run away with the boy and consented to live with him. They were devastated, but they decided to get her married so that she could move on in her life. It was a painful struggle for justice and healing. Her experience highlights how courts perceive acquaintance rape, especially in the case of young girls where their experience of sexual violence is not recognised at all as the abuser was known to the girl.

Sana is the story of the courage and resilience of a father of a young daughter with a physical disability. He narrated his tryst with the CJS and talked about how he and his wife overcame so many health problems that Sana had since her birth and how they accessed healthcare in the city to keep the child alive and healthy. Even her disability was accepted, and she was doing well in a special school until this incident. The apathy of the school and the inability to bribe/grease the system made him decide to not pursue the case in a higher court. He said he had to choose her well-being over punishment for the accused.

Rani was kidnapped, severely assaulted, and raped when she was 16 years old, but she decided to speak herself and narrate her story. Her family migrated to the city from a northern state of India, and they are perceived as outsiders. The boys who kidnapped her had been sexually harassing her for some time. She had raised her voice against them. She described how difficult it was for her parents to register a case of kidnapping against the boys in the first place, followed by their inaction to the hostile environment created in the neighbourhood by the abusers and their families. Despite all evidence, the boys were acquitted. Rani was appalled with the verdict and asked, "If they are not guilty, then am I guilty?"

Anu is a married woman who narrated her story of fighting against her rapist. She was forced to relocate, her husband had to change his office timings, and her life is now about going to court hearing every month and to the police station to complain against the abuse and threats from the abuser, who is out on bail. It has affected her entire family, and she feels guilty about it.

Neeta is a married woman who narrated her ordeal of reporting marital rape. She described her experience of domestic violence for years and her decision to register a case of marital rape. How she was disbelieved at all levels, from the police, to the hospital, to the courts, is vividly described. In court, she was not cross-examined for marital rape, and she felt as though no one even took note of it as they assumed that she was lying. She described the severe impact all this had on her and how she picked up courage and learned all the procedural rigmarole. She wished that her story be read by all so that other women could learn from it and stop abuse in their lives.

The narratives affirm and highlight that multiple interventions and institutional support are required for the survivor and her family, in addition to support from and for facilitating access to police, healthcare, and judicial systems. Survivor-centric changes that have been brought in are related to confidentiality, informed consent, right to treatment, in-camera trials, provision for a support person during court proceedings, and compensation. But the narratives highlight structural injustice that exacerbates the situation for many survivors and their families. The survivor-centric changes, therefore, need to also recognise these structural inequalities and address them to alleviate suffering/reduce adverse impact. It is not just the immediate responses but the continued violations that survivors and their families have to endure that demand attention. Victim compensation represents the state's obligation towards costs for the healing and recovery of the victim.

The narratives starkly note the nature of support that survivors require to be able to go through the CJS. The mere reporting of rape catapults them onto a path of no return, and they have to face uncertainties, humiliation, and repeated visits all in the name of pursuing justice. Aspects such as compensation, shelter homes, counselling, crisis intervention, and support in dealing with the neighbourhood and community seem to take a back seat for them. How to make these relevant and accessible is the challenge. Survivors speak about their lived experiences and also reflect on what needs to change to make this journey less arduous. Those engaged in responding to rape may gain from their experiences and devise ways to reach out and support survivors and their families.

2 "People feel we should always remain sad, not eat well or live well as such an incident has occurred." – Ria's mother

Timeline

The 4-year-old child was brought to the hospital in March 2009 with a history of penile penetration, vaginal bleeding, pain in the abdomen, and pain while walking and passing urine. After the incident, the girl was admitted in the gynaecology ward. The case was closed in one and a half years. The survivor's mother went to court and said that they didn't want to pursue it any further. The judge told them that withdrawal of the case would not have been possible had the incident taken place after the enactment of the new law against child sexual abuse, Protection of Children from Sexual Offences (POCSO) Act in 2012.

Interview conducted with Ria's mother eight
years after the incident

No mother can forget such things. Now also I remember that incident. . . . From where should I start telling you?

This happened one day before Holi when my daughters wanted to go outside to play. It was a happy moment, and I sent my daughters out to play with colours and water. They were wearing tops and slacks/pants that covered the knees. My elder daughter wore a top and leggings, and the younger one was in slacks. I did not feel there was anything wrong in sending them out in leggings. They were both playing out, and I was serving food to my in-laws. After this, I had my food, and when I was cleaning utensils, my elder daughter returned home. When I asked her about Ria, she said, "Ria is playing at *Dada's* place." My daughters called that boy (the abuser) *Dada* (elder brother). So I stood up a little to look in the direction of his house while cleaning utensils – there was soap on my hands. I saw that the door of his house was shut, but I did not sense anything odd (even if the door was shut). I felt it was all right (connoting safety) as she was inside the house, so there was no tension. Had she been playing on the road, then I would have

DOI: 10.4324/9781003281887-3

worried, but as she was in the house, it was okay. So I continued with cleaning and other housework.

After some time, Ria came and told me that she was experiencing a lot of pain (*Mummy khup dukhtay mala*). I scolded her a little by saying, "Why did you go out?" It didn't even occur to me that something like this could have happened. But again, she complained, and pointing to her genitals, she said, "Pain is there." So I made her sit on my lap because she was very small at that time. I asked her to show me where it was painful. I removed her slacks and saw that there was blood on the inner side of her thighs. I was shocked when I saw that and asked her what had happened. Ria told me that she went to Dada's home, and he said to her that he would give her a bag to keep the water balloons and colours to play with. She went inside, and then he did this (*sheput lavla mala sheput* – referring to the penis).

I felt horrible (*kase tari zhale*) and disgusted. I had no balance in my phone, so I took one rupee coin, went to the public booth, and called my husband. I told him to call me on the landline at home. The boy (*Dada*) saw me when I went out as the public booth is next to his house. My husband called on the landline, and I told him the details of what had happened. He immediately came home from work. My father-in-law is very strict, so I didn't tell him anything. I was afraid that he would blame me for what had happened. My husband came back home and saw the blood on Ria's thighs and slacks. Then we informed my in-laws about the incident.

We went to our local doctor and told him about the incident. He immediately understood that something had happened, and he advised us to go to the government hospital and police. The local doctor did not start Ria's treatment. We didn't know what to do, whether to confront him (Dada) directly or not.

We thought that no one would believe us because we had very good relations with the boy's family. He used to come for all meals to my house whenever his mother was out of town. He had grown up in front of us. We knew him since his childhood. He was in twelfth standard at the time of incident, but he was thin and did not look his age.

We decided to go to the police first. The incident had happened in the noon, and we reached the police station between 3:00 to 4:00 p.m. The woman police constable in the police station also checked Ria's genital region and said, "Yes. there is something wrong." We filed the complaint, and the police officer sent some policemen to arrest the boy and brought him to the police station. The boy in the police station denied what he had done. His mother was crying in front of me and said, "Why did you come to the police station? You should have told us before coming here. We would have confronted him." I asked her if she would have believed us at all as any mother would have believed her child. His father had recently brought him a mobile phone, and the boy watched videos (referring to pornography) on it.

When the boy was brought to the police station, the police officer slapped him a couple of times. He was kept in the police station till five in the evening, and then the police got a call from a local corporator[1] who was known to the boy's family. We had returned home when the police called us to say that they were being pressured by the corporator to release the boy. Police told us, "The boy has not done anything, and you were making false allegations." We told the police that he should be punished for what he has done, and now if they want to release him because of the pressure, then that is their look out. We had already filed a police complaint against the boy. Then the police took my statement and took Ria and the boy for a medical check-up to the police hospital.

None of us had eaten anything the entire day. All this while, Ria was not able to urinate. She was telling me that she felt like urinating, but she was not able to sit for it. She did not pass urine for the whole day. The doctor examined her but did not treat her.[2] At the hospital, she was taken inside, and one doctor who was a little old checked her. The doctor informed us that she had been assaulted. After this, the same doctor called the boy inside and slapped him very hard (*sansanit hanli*) and then examined him. By the time the medical got done, it was past midnight. After this, we came back home. The boy must have gotten bail the next day as the police released him. His father passed our house, taking pride in getting his son out of prison on bail. I felt very bad at that time.

The next day, I had to take Ria to a municipal hospital for treatment. She was in extreme pain. There again, the nurse was very rude. When the nurse asked Ria to lie down, she immediately spread her legs, and the nurse remarked, "How many times has this happened with her? Is she used to it?" I retorted, saying that we had come to know today only and that the doctor in the other hospital had asked her to spread her legs for examination. So that's why she may have done it here – spread her legs without being asked to. "Can't you see that she is in pain?"

The municipal hospital carried out all tests, such as sonography, HIV test, and so on. Ria was admitted in the hospital for two days, and a counsellor also met us there. We were asked by the hospital to pay for tests. I don't recall the amount, but the counsellor intervened to waive the fees. Ria was on medications and saline. Once she passed urine, she felt better and was able to move around. She was in pain for two to three days.

The municipal hospital had informed the police about the incident, so we received a call from the police. The police questioned our visit to the municipal hospital. They wondered if we did not trust them as we had again reported the incident to a municipal hospital. We clarified that we had come to the hospital for treatment as the doctor at the police hospital had not treated Ria.

The case went on for a year. We went for two to three hearings. Later, I was called by the court, but I could not go. I don't travel alone anywhere. My husband works as a driver, so for every court hearing, he had to take leave, which meant losing his wages for the day. We could not afford this as he is the only earning member. Many people advised us that we should take money from the boy's family and settle the case. But we told all of them that "our daughter is not for sale (*amhi amchi mulgi kai vikayala kadhali ka*)." We told them that we did not want a single rupee.

Also, my in-laws started saying that Ria was growing up. She had to hear those words again and again. She has also not forgotten the incident. She sometimes mentions to me, "They used to stay here," so she still remembers. She was very small at that time, but still, she has not forgotten the incident. Every time we went out, she felt it was for the *case*. The boy's lawyer also advised us to take the case back as the boy was not getting a job anywhere due to a criminal case against him. We then thought that he has been punished enough and also decided to focus on our daughter's future and take back the case.

The boy's lawyer asked us to give a written statement that we misunderstood the incident at that time and there was no sexual violence. I told the lawyer, "I will not lie at all." My daughter had gone to the boy's house, and she told me such an incident had taken place. I refused to lie in the court. So the boy's lawyer said, "Do what you want to do."

We went to court and requested for withdrawal of the case. There was a male judge who asked us if anybody was pressuring us to take the case back. I told the judge that we were not being pressured but were concerned about our daughter having to hear the same things again and again. This happened in court in 2014.

The judge also told me that if the incident had taken place after two to three years, it would not have been possible for us to withdraw the case. There was a new stringent law against child sexual abuse that did not allow any complainant to withdraw their case.

It took a long time for the case to come up for hearing in court (it took one year per the current procedures). If the case had come up sooner, we would have done something to punish the boy. The delay led to a lot of talk and speculation in the community about whether we had withdrawn the complaint. If the case is true, why so much delay? People around felt that we should always remain sad and not eat well or live well as such an incident had occurred. Is that possible?

The people living around us started blaming us for going to the police. They alleged that we had made a false allegation. They all stopped talking with us. Later, I heard that the boy's cousin also got into some trouble. The family again tried to get support from the local party office, but the party told them to leave this place. Eventually, the boy's family relocated to another place.

The boy's parents were good; they were not bad people. They did not want to stay here and left this area. But even after they left from here, people in the area did not behave properly around us. If there is any programme organised in the area, they will not call us, and will not speak to us. So I constantly feel as if I have done something wrong. We often feel we should not have filed the complaint and should have left the matter there itself. My daughter was able to walk properly (meaning no serious harm was caused).

People around us really bother us. Had they dealt with it maturely, it would have helped us to overcome this. Why would anyone lie about such an incident? We were not invited for any function, including pooja (prayer), in the area and my mother-in-law (MIL) would get very upset.

I will tell you about another incident in the neighbourhood. One woman living close by used to throw garbage in front of our house. My father-in-law (FIL) or I would clean it, but we knew that she was doing it deliberately. One day I got angry, and I picked up all that garbage and kept it near her house. It triggered off a quarrel between us, and she referred to the incident that took place with Ria.

She said, "That boy made your daughter bleed from her anus, but you were not able to do anything (*Tuzhya mulichya gandicha rakta kadhala tari tu kahi nahi karu shaklis*), and when I threw garbage, you have thrown it back in front of my house." Then she went on to accuse me of taking money from the boy's family. I told her, "We have not taken any money from anyone, and we will starve to death but not take money." I also told her to go to court and find out herself about the case. But I felt very bad at that time as she used such foul language. I kept calm and spoke politely to her. I told her that we were concerned about our daughter and did not want her to suffer, and so we withdrew the case. It's been so many years since the incident, but this neighbour still referred to that incident, and even now, if we have any guests or anyone asking for our address, this lady tells them about what happened to our daughter.

People come to our home and ask us if this has happened to our child? I deliberately deny it, as what's the point in talking about it repeatedly? I feel like my daughter is being abused again and again (*khapli kadhlya sarakhe* – not letting the injury heal). Now, as the case is closed, I feel that everything is over, and we do not want to talk about it anymore. I have torn all the papers related to the case. My husband was upset with me and told me that we should always keep the proof with us. I know that what he said was right, but I said I want to erase all bad memories. The file of the case used to be there at home, and the girls would take it out and read the papers. So I just tore everything.

I had a lot of respect for the police. I used to feel very proud of them and aspired to join the police force. When the incident where the woman from our area threw garbage in front of my house abused me and my daughter, I had called the police to complain about the woman. But they did not take any action and just ignored the complaint. So I told the senior police official that I wanted to join the police force, but after seeing the behaviour of the police, I am glad I did not (*mazhi iccha meleye police vyayachi*). The police are always on the side of the wrong people. In general, we expect that police will give justice, but in reality, nothing happens like that.

My son was born after this incident, so he does not know anything. My elder daughter knows everything, but we have kept her in our native place. Due to the attitude of the neighbours, we were forced to send our elder daughter to my parents' home in the village. My elder daughter is very quiet. Even if someone slaps her, she will not utter a single word. Therefore, I am concerned about her safety, and so I have kept her in the village. We miss her, but we felt that sending her to our native place was the best for her as she is safe. She will be in the village till she finishes her tenth exam. She is about one and a half years older than Ria. But she still remembers everything. Ria has vague memory, but she has not forgotten the people in the boy's house. We also will never forget them. We didn't talk to her about what had happened. For almost two to three months, whoever came to visit us would talk about the incident. So she heard it again and again, but later we stopped talking about it. Then she forgot everything slowly. We did not force her to forget it, but she forgot it.

Ria has become very smart now. If someone says anything to her, she gives it back – she retorts (*Jar hila koni aare kele na tar ti lagech kare karte*). After the incident, I did not allow Ria to go out of the house. She was 4.5 years old at the time of incident. Since then, I have not allowed her to go out, only to school, class, and home.

She is in seventh standard now and goes alone to school as it is nearby. My daughter feels that I am a very bad mother as I don't let her go out. Now, how do I explain this to her? I do say that people outside are bad, so I cannot send her out alone. If I am working inside the house, I don't let her go out at all. She keeps arguing with me over this and tells me how other girls are allowed to go out and wear whatever they want. But I just say that she can do whatever she wants when she grows up as an adult, but not now.

My husband had informed my parents about the incident, who kept it to themselves and told me not to disclose it to my brother. But my parents said, "I don't look after the girls or keep an eye on them." The boy's family was so close to us, and my daughters would often go to their house, spend time there, and change clothes there. It never occurred to me that something like this could ever happen.

But it is good that the boy's family moved out of this place. If they had continued to live here, we would have never been able to forget the incident. The boy's family was not in touch with us directly but kept sending us messages through relatives to withdraw the case. The boy kept saying that he had not done anything and that my daughter might have gotten injured by his nails. I said, "But why did your nails even reach there (the girl's genitals)?"

Recently, we received news from some relative that the boy was very sick and vomited blood. We felt that he had been punished for what he has done.

Notes

1   A local corporator is a person who is a member of a local governing body.
2   The police had taken Ria to the police hospital per their procedures. The police hospital is known to restrict themselves to examination and evidence collection. It does not provide treatment to rape survivors. This has been documented by CEHAT through an intervention study (Contractor, S., Divekar, R., and Rajan, A. (2000). Report on observations conducted at the police hospital. Centre for Enquiry into Health and Allied Themes 2010).

3 "Do whatever you want to do. As a father, I will not take back the case." – Sara's father

Timeline

A six-year-old girl was brought to a municipal hospital at 11:45 p.m. and examined immediately. She came with a history of touching and fingering by a known person in the public toilet and later in her house. Her parents went to work, so the girl didn't tell them about the incident but complained of stomach pain. The mother gave her a tablet as she thought it was due to the consumption of too many sweets. Later, when the boy abused her in their house, the girl showed her mother blood-stained underwear which she had hidden. A medical examination found scratch marks, injuries in the genital region, and redness six days after the assault. The Juvenile Justice Board had closed the case as the boy was a minor, and the maximum length of punishment is three years.

Interview with Sara's father seven years after the incident

Sara was alone in the home at that time. She had returned from school and was about to change her clothes. That is when the boy came in and asked her for water. He entered the house and locked the door from inside. My son came home and thought the mother was there inside. He peeped from the window and saw that this boy was there in our house. My son said, "Open the door or I will beat you." At that time, my son was also young. Now he is 18 years old. He shouted, but the boy (abuser) pushed my son and ran away. The boy was there inside the house for a long time.

My daughter started crying and told my son, "Dada, he did this to me. He forcefully closed my mouth. . . . He did this to me" (*aisa* referring to the specific act). We (parents of Sara) were out for work and were not aware of the incident. When we came back home, we planned to take Sara to the hospital. Everybody told us to first lodge a complaint, but when we went there, the police asked us to take her first to the municipal hospital. The doctor looked at my daughter and asked us to go to the bigger municipal hospital.

DOI: 10.4324/9781003281887-4

Sara was admitted to the ICU in the bigger municipal hospital for a few days. The police came there and recorded statements but did not give us any paper. We didn't get the help we needed from the police and the hospital. The police caught the boy as an eyewash and was kept in custody for two days and was then released. I again lodged a complaint against him. After that, he was caught, kept in an observation home for two to three days, and was again released from there as well.

The boy (referring to the abuser) lived in our neighbourhood and is a (drug) addict (*Gardulla*). He used to take drinks and do *nasha* (ganja, charas). He came to Sara's school two to three times and threatened her. The police arrested him, and he was kept in the boarding (observation home) for two to three days. He was almost 18 years old; two to three days remained until he turned 18. He was then released.

The boy and his father troubled us a lot. His father threatened me, saying, "If you don't take back the case, we will kill you. You have destroyed my son's life. . . . My son was going to start a government job." I only said, "Look at what you have done to my daughter, and you are fighting with me? I will complain about this, and you can do whatever you want to. Do you want to murder me? Do that, bring whoever you want to bring." In order to suppress the case, the abuser and his family pressured us a lot. I also approached a few people, but we did not get the kind of help we needed.

Firstly, the police were not taking our FIR. The police had come when Sara was admitted to the hospital in the ICU. We told the police all that had happened. Police noted all that, prepared some papers, but did not give us any paper. We asked them for the paper and told them that we wanted to file FIR. They said, "Your FIR is already recorded, and you will get the copy later." But they did not give us any copy.

After discharge from the municipal hospital, we took Sara to a private doctor as she was still suffering. We did not receive proper treatment from the municipal hospital. She had pain in her stomach. The treatment at the municipal hospital was not useful, so we had to go to a private doctor. The private doctor treated Sara well, but even now sometimes she has problems. So we have to give her medicines. She is 12 years old now but still sometimes complains of stomachache and feels dizzy (*Sir ghumne lagta hai*). She doesn't go out to play with anyone because of fear.

After Sara's treatment, I spoke to my wife. I said, "Let our daughter go to school and continue her education." She is studying, and this incident should not spoil her future. Even now, I feel she should continue to go to school, but she won't go. Every now and then, she does not want to go to school. She is very scared. If any boy says anything, she immediately runs away from the school.

I am a driver. My wife is a domestic worker and washes utensils in house-holds. We drop the children to school in the morning, and in the afternoon, Sara comes back home on her own. Earlier, my son and Sara would go and come back together, but now my son has left school. He is taking his exams outside school. So now my son drops Sara to school in the morning, and she comes back on her own in the afternoon at twelve o'clock. She is in the seventh standard now and is average in her studies. Before, she was good at her studies, but then after that incident, she did not go to school for a month or two. The treatment also took some time. She used to experience pain at 3:00 a.m. All this used to create a problem for her regular schooling. Then even we thought let the school take a back seat for some time as Sara's health is more important.

My in-laws stay next door. They were also not at home at the time of the incident. Their house was locked, and the boy took advantage of this (*Usne chance mara*). Not many people in our area know about the incident, and only our neighbours are aware. They (neighbours) stopped talking to my daughter. Earlier, we used to go to their houses. But after the incident, our visits decreased. The abuser has political connections, and he uses them to threaten everybody. He also comes to collect *hafta* (extortion) in that area, so people are afraid of him. There are people from a western Indian state in our area, and they do "gold work" (*Sone ka kaam*). That boy comes to col-lect money from them, and nobody from the neighbourhood says anything against him.

The boy and his father started threatening me, saying, "Take back the case, or else we will murder you." The case was heard in juvenile justice court, but he was released. I went to court two to three times and used to have fights with the abuser and his companions. The abuser used to be accompanied by many people in court.

My daughter had to go to court as well. They took my daughter inside and made her stand in front of the judge, closed the door, and started asking her questions. The judge asked her, "What happened? How did it happen?" My daughter told the judge everything. They allowed the mother inside, and then they called me as well and asked me questions like "When did you come to know about it?" I said, "When I came to know about the incident, I left my work and came home." Then I was asked, "Then what was the first thing you did?"

The judge sentenced the abuser and gave him some punishment. But we don't know what punishment was given to the boy. So it was all over in two to three days, but they didn't give us any order. The boy was released after a few days. We don't know whether he was released on bail or not. What the court decided in the case was not explained to us. Thus, our court experience was not good. We did not meet any lawyer; no lawyer even came to speak with us. No one explained anything to me or my daughter. We had a public prosecutor (PP). I know he is supposed to be our lawyer. But it is known to all that these lawyers (PPs) don't do anything. I am sure there is some kind of understanding/settlement between the PP and the private lawyer. They are all lawyers, and they know each other very well. And nobody knows us (the complainant and her family). They have been working together for several years, so they mutually decide on how to proceed in a case.

My wife fought with the defence lawyer when he was using "dirty words" (*ganda shabd*). He asked my daughter and also my wife, "Did he remove clothes, and then what did he (abuser) do?" He was asking a whole lot of questions. My wife said, "Whatever it was we have told the police and the hospital people, they know it better, what happened and what did not. How can you ask such questions to us?" He said, "It is our job to ask all this, if there were clothes on the girl's body or not. What happened? What did he do? We need to ask all these things." Sara was such a small girl at that time. Should anyone ask such questions to a small girl?

Then it is but obvious that our daughter would start crying there only, in front of the judge, "Mummy, I don't like it, and they are asking me such questions. I am feeling very dirty. They are asking me such questions." I said to judge, "Sir, I do not want to do anything. Whatever it is you have to do, whatever the report is, it is in front of you, okay? I do not want to say anything about it." I said, "It is in your hands whether to put him in jail or set him free."

But the abuser's lawyer was good. He had taken INR 10,000–12,000, so he was acting smart (*jada ud raha tha*). He asked my wife, "What was the first thing you saw? Then who filed the complaint? Who peeped from the window? Then who saw that boy? It can be someone else also." My wife argued with him and said, "My son is not a kid." And when he peeped from the window, he called out for opening the door. At that time, abuser only came out of the house and ran away. Otherwise, my son would have surely beaten him up. And both were of the same age then, but the abuser pushed my son aside and ran away.

My wife was upset with all this, and her concern was that other people from our native place and relatives would come to know about the case, and then who would marry our daughter? So even I said, "Okay, we won't go. Even if the judge calls, we will not go because of such questions . . . but we will not take the case back."

We went to court for a month, and after that, the boy was released. They did not call me to court. The judge said, "You need not come to the court, and we will take the required action against him."

We have seen that boy around in our area. He has married a girl from our area, so he comes regularly. We often come across him, and he is always drunk. We don't interact with him as he is always ready to pick up a fight. We just ignore him. There is no point in fighting with him as there is no one to support us. Even the police are supporting the abuser, and no one is there to support us, so we don't talk with him. He threatens me, and I listen to it; that's it. Let them do whatever they want; we will see what to do.

That boy has been giving us so much trouble that sometimes we feel that we should relocate to another place. Right now, I don't have a copy of the police complaints I made for threats; otherwise, I would have shown them to you. I just complained a few days back again. So either he should be arrested or some investigation should be done, but nothing happens.

Recently there was a fight between the abuser and my son. I saw them fighting in a garden. They were beating each other. I went inside the garden and slapped that boy. After that, I called the police by using my phone, but that boy ran away from there. When the police came, they said, "You are making us come here for the same thing. Don't you know we have other duties?"

The father of the boy says that his son is not getting a government job as there is a criminal case against him. There are other criminal charges against the boy as well, like theft, robbery, and drug use. The boy was caught by police many times due to all these other charges, but his father says that the charges made by us are severe (*bada case hai*), so we should take them back.

A few days back, the boy's father sent someone who offered money to *settle* the case. The person told me to withdraw the case as it's been many years now, and so there is no point in continuing it. I told him that I will not withdraw this case. I know no one is helping us now, but maybe someone will help us tomorrow. He offered us INR 100,000 and was willing to go upto INR 150,000 or even double it.

The boy's father has been consistently using his political connections to threaten me over phone and say, "Come to this place or we will kidnap your son." I go wherever they call me. They make me sit alone and meet some people. Those people tell me, "See, you should not blow these things out of proportion (*Baat badhane ke nahi hota hai*). You will also be defamed in all this. Make some money if you want, settle the matter (*Mandvali*), and leave him alone."

Thus, I feel there is a need to change the police system because they accept money and settle cases like this. Due to this, people like us are suffering (*hum jaise log aise hi maar rahe hai*). People who have money are powerful (*bade log hai*), and they have their "setting" (refers to a settlement). In our case also, the boy's family gave money, and their son was out. We kept "standing" (means waiting for justice) with papers in our hands to be heard, but there was nobody to listen to us.

The abuser and his family were born here, so they know many people here. We are from a northern state of India. Who is going listen to us here? (They are migrants.) This also makes a difference – the locals have more influence. And we are from another state. The police didn't move the case ahead. During the trial, the police officer who was handling the case also expired. So the case was handed over to another officer, and this new officer did not show any interest. When we received the call from the police station, then it was all our work; they did not take any responsibility. All such matters are settled by taking money.

All these problems forced me to resign from my job. I was working in an airline company for two years but had resigned from this good job as I had to take several days of leave for the case. The repeated visits to the police station, juvenile justice court, and the hospital compelled me to do this. After that, I have not been able to find that kind of job. The job at the airline was good; it was only for eight hours, and there was time to do other things as well. I used to get a monthly salary of INR 6,000 at that time. Now I drive a tourist car. So I have to go outstation for two to three days and also the work is not fixed. We had to spend a lot of money on Sara's treatment in the private hospital. Even for the court visit, I had to take Sara, as my wife is not educated, so she does not know much. I am also not educated, but then I had to go everywhere to understand what was happening in the case. I am the only earning person in the family. My son goes for tuition from 3:00 p.m. to 8:00 p.m., and after that, he sits at home and studies. I have the entire responsibility of the family, and in today's time, with so much inflation, it is so difficult to manage.

My wife also said if the police are not listening to us, then we will approach a lawyer who can then take the matter to a higher court. She was working as a maid at this lawyer's home. We were worried about the cost as following up on a case means loss of wages for me. If I will not go to work, then how will I run the house (*Ghar nahi chalega*)? (He will not be able to manage expenses.)

Once or twice, when I tried to follow up on the case, the abuser and his family fought with my son. They assaulted my son with a blade (*Vaar kia tha*), and he suffered a deep cut. My wife went and registered a complaint against the boy. Then again, the police suppressed the matter. He has not yet harmed me, but he threatened me. I said, "Do whatever you want to do, but I will not take the case back." The conditions earlier were not good. At that time, I was no one in front of you, but now certainly I have built up my courage and will stand up against them. I will get the father arrested and his son also.

The boy who did this with Sara also did it with another girl. The girl was from another area, so he kidnapped her, and this case was also going on against the boy. We brought this to the notice of the police, but they said, "Let it go. You focus on your case. Don't tell us about other cases." I said, "He has done this to another girl also, and so I am informing you."

So it is a clear thing how the law is! Now look – the one (victim) who should have got justice did not get it, and the culprit is roaming freely and keeps threatening us that if we don't take the case back, they will show us. Even we are afraid. My son goes out alone, and if they do anything to him, then . . . He is our only son.

Because of this, we are keeping mum and not doing anything. I told my son that if he spots them, then he should change direction and take another road. If they are sitting someplace, he should not go there. My son is a little bit hot-headed. He says, "Papa, I will not say anything on my own, but now if he comes, I will not leave him."

The problem with the legal system is that the one who needs justice does not get it. I always wonder that so much happened to my daughter and us, and that boy still drinks, does drugs, and threatens us even now.

4 "We had to choose between education and well-being of our daughter versus appeal in the higher court." – Sana's father

Sana, a 16-year-old deaf and mute girl, was brought by police to the hospital in December 2012 at 5:00 a.m. She was examined at 7:30 a.m. One day before, at 3:00 p.m., she was abducted by two unknown men, and when she resisted, they inflicted injuries with a blade on her upper limbs. The abusers used a condom. The abuse continued for a few hours. Sana returned home at 6:30 p.m. and informed her mother about the incident. The family went to the police station, and she was brought to the hospital at 5:00 a.m. The men were acquitted, and the family decided not to appeal in a higher court. The court said that there was no adequate evidence to prove that the boys were guilty. When contacted for the research study, the father was happy that someone was concerned for them and spoke at length.

Interview with Sana's father conducted four years and one month after the incident

Whatever happened was a bad dream, and we want to forget about it. And now we want to focus on Sana's education and her future. That is also the reason why we did not appeal in a higher court as the continuation of the case was a hindrance (*badha*) in Sana's education. The main problem is in our system; one has to make multiple visits to several places and follow up for everything (*bahut bhagna padta hai*). Further, the loopholes/rigmaroles (*chakke panje*), such as "This is required," "That is required," and "This has to be done this way," in all this a lot of time gets wasted. The main focus should be the child and her future.

So we decided not to appeal in a higher court. If we had appealed in a higher court, then I am confident that we would have won the case. But it would have no meaning. The punishment to the boy would not have benefited Sana (*Usko saja mil gayi ya iska labh ho gaya, aisa kuch nahi hota*). Over the years, his family has also become very polite, and they apologised to us as well. So we decided not to appeal in a higher court.

DOI: 10.4324/9781003281887-5

As Sana is already deaf and mute, and so her education is very important. We brought a full stop to all this matter, as the court said there is no solid (*pakka*) evidence.

I am sure the abuser had done it. He always used to follow these girls on the local bus that they took to go to school and everywhere. We knew about him as Sana had told us that there was one boy who followed her. He did this, so why did he do this (non-verbal actions to show that he touched her)?

When we used to accompany Sana to school, he would not come. But when we did not go, he would take that chance and used to go on the bus. That day, it was the festival of Gokulasthami. Their school had called the students to make them understand the meaning of the festival. So she went for the program, but it did not last for a long time. On her way back home, that boy somehow convinced her to come with him. He knew that Sana loved vada pav and brought her to the railway station and gave her vada pav. The boy then took Sana to a bridge at the backside of the railway station. There he called another boy. He was also named in the complaint. We did not know what had happened. When Sana came home, she started crying. She did not understand what happened to her and was not able to articulate the incident. Later, she also told me that about fifteen to twenty days before this incident also, these boys had attacked her.

During that incident, these boys took my daughter forcibly inside a public toilet. Suddenly one lady came there to the public toilet. I don't know who that lady was, but when she came inside the toilet, Sana set herself free from there. She came home and again started screaming a lot (*Aakrosh*). Her mother asked what happened, but she was not able to tell us. After the incident that happened on the bridge, we took Sana to the police station. There was a social worker in the police station who spoke to her inside a room and enquired in detail, and then we came to know what happened. Then the boy's sketch was drawn according to the description given by her, and based on that, he was arrested and was kept inside the lockup. Sana also told police about the second boy who was caught later.

First, we went to the police station. Police informed us that medical evidence was required in this case, so we went to a municipal hospital. In the municipal hospital, the experience was good. Sana was admitted for three to four days. She was given treatment, and all reporting about the incident was done in a form filled by a doctor. She had injuries on her hands, so medicines were given and the course was completed.

After discharge from the municipal hospital, we went to the police station. Sana was shown the photograph of the boy and was again asked to identify him correctly. After the boys were arrested by police, they took Sana to identify the spot where this had happened. In order to ascertain if she was telling the truth, they took her to other places also (to confuse her). But she was able to identify the spot.

At the police station, the boys confessed to what they had done, but the police could not prove it in court (*Police sabit nahi kar payi*). The police again asked for medical examination (*medical ka claim rakha*) and informed us that the reports from the municipal hospital could be wrong. The police then took Sana to the police hospital. The medical reports of the hospital indicated that such a thing (rape) had happened. Then the police started asking who had seen the incident and if anyone had seen it (crime). We said no, there was no eyewitness. So on that basis, the boys were acquitted after the case went on for a year in a sessions court.

If you see in my case, the police behaved quite well with me. They did all that was required, but there was some hanky-panky going on within the police department (*police ne kuch to gadbad ki*). Due to this, we lost the case, although it was strong.

During the court trial, four lawyers were changed in one year. The first lawyer was very good and worked really hard to get the case on the board. But the last lawyer was not so good. Those boys had a lot of money and had hired well-known lawyers. My daughter was called in court ten to fifteen times. My wife was also called in court. Being a father, it was not easy for me then and now. I am controlling myself while I am talking to you. But being a mother, my wife broke down in court. The court was then adjourned for ten minutes. There has been no change in our judiciary system even after the Nirbhaya incident. The mockery of all this was that even while this case was going in session court, the defence lawyers were appealing in high court.

The boys did not get bail, so they were in jail for a year. This is what I know, but what may have happened actually one doesn't know (meaning that was told by the police may be less than the truth). One boy was living close to our house, but the other was in another area. We were called again and again in court. When Sana was called to give a statement, then they also called the teacher. When the teacher went inside the court, my wife was not allowed to be with Sana. It was the teacher, the judge, and the lawyers from both sides. I feel that at least one of the parents should have been allowed inside the courtroom. Later, the teacher was called separately three times when my daughter was not there. The court also called the other girls from the school. Those girls told how that boy was following them and teasing Sana. All due process and steps were neatly followed by the court. Yet the final decision of the court was that there was no evidence. I did not take a copy of the order. I planned to take it out for appeal in the higher court, but the behaviour of the school changed our decision. The school authorities started saying that our daughter was spoiling the name of the school. The principal was bad (*badmaash*), and they troubled us for two and a half months. They said, "The school has a name, and we have done so much for these children (deaf and mute). But because of your daughter, the school's prestige is being affected." I asked them, "Should you be sympathetic towards my daughter or blame her? How can you treat her like this?" The school responded, "We are doing what we can. Otherwise, you can send her to another school and can appear for exams from elsewhere." Can you imagine? That they even made such a suggestion. I heard it all, but then they also realised that this was not correct. However, the school authorities took all kinds of things in writing from us. They took an undertaking that we will be responsible if anything happens to our daughter, and we will drop her and pick her up from school every day. We had no choice, so we did that. My wife used to go every day to school with Sana.

This was after the case was over at the sessions court. When the case was going on, they did not allow her to attend school. They said, "She cannot come to school till the case is going on in court." So she was at home for two years. She failed last year, so she lost that year, and in the second year also, she suffered in school due to harassment by schoolteachers. They would keep asking her, "Why did you speak to that boy, and what were you doing with him? Why did that boy come near you?" But we still fought it out, and we explained saying that this boy would follow her to the bus, he is a rogue (*badmaash*), and so they also understood. They heard us out and said, "We will look into it," but kept instructing us to be careful and insisted that someone accompany her to school to prevent such an incident again. For the safety of my daughter, my wife was going every day with her. But now I said we would not do this. If we continue to do, it then it will be wrong, and I had to take a stand to stop this.

My daughter had a bad time, and we want to consider it as a bad dream and forget about it. I had come to Dilaasa in the hospital once but could not locate it during that visit and never came back. Now I wish I had so that we would have some support. See, whatever has to happen in someone's life, it is bound to happen. If any help or support is destined, then it is bound to be received. My wife is a housewife, and I work at an institute. Sana has been dumb and deaf, and we have had to put in a lot of effort not just during the two years since the incident but right from her birth as her health was critical. She is our fourth daughter, and her condition was critical for three to four months after her birth. She was diagnosed with rickets when she was 6 months old, and we discovered that she could not hear when she was 1 year old.

We met good doctors who referred us to hospitals that provided low-cost treatment. We were not eligible for free services as I had a government job. But our financial condition was not good, so we struggled to get her therapy and hearing aid. We looked after her very well. Once we got her a hearing aid, we were able to secure her admission to school. She was good at her studies. She adjusted well in school, and then when she was in eighth standard, this happened (incident of sexual violence). She is good at drawing. She says that she will grow up to become a drawing teacher. She takes private tuitions for drawing, and she has passed with flying colours. Her drawing teacher is very proud of her.

She will appear for tenth this year. Let me show you pictures of her drawings. (Sana's father showed pictures of her sketches. He explained each of them with pride.) She was awarded INR 6,000 in a drawing competition one and a half years back. Sana now teaches students who are appearing for the examination of elementary drawing. She has drawn a portrait of an actress too – Priyanka Chopra. This year we did not allow her to pursue any activity. Now kids are kids – you (signaling to the interviewers) are also mothers, so you would know . . . but we have to push our kids. She is very sincere and is serious about her studies. She puts an alarm on my mobile and wakes up early to study. She got 78% in eighth standard. But due to this tension, she got affected. The school environment is not good and supportive. A teacher is God's second form (*dusra roop*), so it is not good to say anything negative about teachers. But I think the school authorities are also discriminating (*jaatiwaadi*) based on our religion (Muslim). They harass her a lot through repeated questioning. They did not allow her to give her tenth exams and said she was not ready as she would not score well. We were willing to send her for extra coaching, but they did not agree. My daughter's one more year got wasted. Now all her classmates have been promoted to the next standard. Sana feels like she is cornered and wonders why. Sometimes she also feels that she is not capable. She has one more health problem – her eyes keep watering (he then showed how her eyes don't close [completely]). There is a problem with the tear gland, and her tears don't collect at all.

Whatever it is I feel that God has given us a flower which does not have a fragrance, but we have to take care of it and look after it. We have to accept her as she is and support her in the best way possible.

I would like to mention that a lot needs to change in our system. When such an incident takes place, who the person is should be considered. If the person is abled (*sudhrud*) or above 16 years old or a normal person, then she should go through a process. But this is a person with a disability, we should consider what she is going through. We need to bring change regarding this. (He was referring to the process and procedures to be friendly to persons with disabilities.)

Also, whether the accused confesses in the police station, or in court, or in front of a crowd, that should be accepted, right? That did not happen in our case. It is the most painful thing. Till the end, we thought that we would win the case. The boys were kept in jail and were given jail clothes and token numbers. My daughter identified them in court through videoconferencing. Is this not enough evidence?

So why this is not recognised by law? So many such criminals will get away. In our case, all steps were followed, but I feel that somewhere the justice chain was interfered with. It started well with a good public prosecutor who explained everything to us and was good. But later, the boys hired well-known criminal lawyers, and then things changed. A new public prosecutor came, then she disappeared, and then another one came. Then even she went, and a new one came. So what I feel is *Tum mere se nahi pate, baju hatao, tum bhi nahi pate . . . jo pati usse kaam karaya* (It's possible that the defence lawyers were trying to make some underhand dealing with the public prosecutor and kept asking for change until they were able to strike a deal). This is what I feel.

Having gone through the court procedure, I feel there should be someone in court who can help people like us. It is important that a person has complete knowledge and can understand all aspects of the case. Someone who knows the CJS and aware of the rights of the victim and accused and also knows how the accused and his lawyers operate.

The police were okay with us. See, the current state of affairs is that if I don't get something (not receiving a bribe), I will not do anything – whether you are a social worker or a judge or any ordinary person or beggar. See, no one asked for it (bribe) – I will not lie. I am hungry, but I am feeling shy to ask for it, but you are cooking, and you ask me, "Do you want it?" Then even if I did not ask for it, still I get it from somewhere. There was a police officer – he was going to retire in a few months, so he managed it like that (referring to the police officer having taken a bribe from the accused).

The day we heard the order in the court, we were very angry with the judge. Nothing was read out; they just spoke in English. The judge dictated to the typist, and it was typed, and both the boys started dancing happily. When we came out, their *chacha-kaka* (uncles) of the boys came and said, "Whatever has happened cannot be changed, but now don't take it ahead (meaning don't pursue the case), please – it will only create problems for us and you also." So I said okay. We had tried to hire a private lawyer, but he said it was too late now. Nothing can be done and can only be sent for appeal in a higher court. Then we saw the attitude of the school, which turned bad (*khatta nikla*). So then we thought that there was no point in pursuing the case. We have to nurture this plant, and if we are giving too much water to it with the hope that it will grow fast, then that will not happen. So if we now go for appeal in a higher court, and if her education is affected, what is the use?

For example, if a rich man is walking on the street and someone attacks him and demands money, then what will the man do? Will he keep his money or his life? He will hand over his money only, right? Why will he give up his life? So that is what I thought – education is more important. Sending those boys to jail has no meaning, and whether they will be reformed or not, who knows. There was another case against him, someone told me – that boy is again in jail for a similar case, so this is what it is. So for them, committing crimes has become their habit. Once they have been set free, they feel they can commit more crimes and get away easily.

5 "Every time there was a new lawyer, I was called again, and I was asked the same thing again and again." – Bindu's mother

Bindu, 16 years old, came to the hospital at 2:43 p.m. and was examined at 2:50 p.m. in August 2014. The incident took place forty-five days ago. The abuser was a 22-year-old boy who had proposed to Bindu in the past, but she had declined, which he did not like. On the day of the incident, he drugged her through a drink and took her to his house and raped her. The next day, he took her to his aunt's house in another city, where she was raped every day by the abuser and compelled to do all household chores. After this, Bindu was brought back to Mumbai, and the abuse continued. It was only when she threatened suicide that the abuser called Bindu's mother. Bindu's parents had filed a missing complaint, and so the local corporator called them to the police station, and the police were informed that the girl and boy knew each other and had run away. The local corporator misguided the police at the behest of the abuser. Bindu did not tell her mother about the abuse as she was in a state of shock and was unable to tell her parents about the abuse she had suffered. Police didn't take Bindu to a hospital for a medical examination, and her parents also didn't realise that she should be taken to the hospital. So the parents, along with Bindu, went home. But after two days, Bindu fell unconscious at home and was taken to the nearest public hospital. The doctors at the public hospital told the parents to take Bindu to a higher health facility. The police were informed by the hospital about the abuse that happened with Bindu, and an FIR was filed two days after the medico-legal examination of Bindu.

Interview with Bindu's mother three years after the incident

Bindu has been married for two months now. Before marriage, we informed everything to the boy's family about the incident. Bindu's husband works in an NGO. This NGO works in the area where we live. They provide financial aid to people for services, such as marriage or death rites. They had helped me in this case (rape) also. The people from the NGO suggested to us that

DOI: 10.4324/9781003281887-6

we get her married to someone who is known so that Bindu would not have any tension after marriage.

There is a local corporator (Nagar Sevak) in my area. I got a call from his office on 13th of August because I had distributed Bindu's photographs and given my number when we were searching for her. I got a call at 1:00 p.m. and was called into his office. When I went there, the boy's mother was sitting there. I was told that my daughter had been at her home for the last two days. I scolded the boy's mother and said, "I have a copy of the missing complaint with me. My daughter has been missing for the last one and a half months, and how is she saying that she was with her for two days?" But the local corporator advised me to settle the matter (*idhar hi mandvali kar*). But I said, "Whoever you are, whether you are a local corporator or a big minister, whatever happens, the matter will be sorted out in the police station only." I told him to get my daughter to the police station in half an hour.

The boy's mother used to work in a beer bar, and the boy was working as part of an orchestra (*dhol bajaneka kaam karta tha*) in the area. His work was to play the drums (*dhol*) at weddings or festivals. During one such festival, he saw Bindu, who was at the event with her grandmother. He behaved inappropriately with her and tried to touch her. Bindu slapped him, and that was what he kept in his mind. He started keeping an eye on Bindu and found out where she lived. She was living with my MIL (mother-in-law) at the time of the incident. As she wanted to learn tailoring, she used to go for tailoring classes. My MIL always accompanied her wherever she went. But that day, my MIL was unwell, so my daughter asked her if it was okay if she went alone for her tailoring class as it was just across the road. It was afternoon. That boy had kept track of Bindu, and the moment he saw her alone, he and his friend kidnapped her. His friend was not arrested but was called as a witness. Can you imagine, the one who was with him that day was called as a witness to support his case? The police said they could not include many names in the FIR.

When Bindu was found almost one and a half months after filing a missing complaint, she couldn't disclose about abuse as she was in a state of shock. The police wrote something on a paper and told us to go. Just when we were leaving the police station at 2:00 a.m., one police officer came out and told us to take Bindu to the hospital. But he did not explain why we should go to the hospital. Also, it did not occur to me that she needed to be taken to a doctor. Ideally, the police should have taken her to the hospital for a medical check-up after she had been found. This is what they are supposed to do in all cases of kidnapping. When we reached home, Bindu started complaining of stomach pain. So in the morning, I took her to the police station as I did not want to go to the hospital without the police. But it was on Independence Day, so the police said they wouldn't be able to accompany us to the hospital. We did not know that the police should have taken us to the hospital. We went to a public hospital on our own.

Bindu was examined at the hospital. I did not want to be present during her check-up as she was screaming in pain. But the doctor told me that I have to be present. There were two to three lady doctors who conducted her examination. They used some instruments, and no man was present. When the doctor was examining her genitals, Bindu told the doctor that she was raped. Her genital area was infected, she complained of itching all over her body, and her skin was peeling (*chamdi chamdi nikal rahi thi*).

Her genital area was badly infected. The doctor told me that she would give me the report and that I should go to the police station. So I learned about what had happened only when she went in for the examination and told the doctor. I took her aside and asked her what had happened. She told me what had happened and how the boy used to come in the night, and she was unaware of what he did to her. The doctor gave us the report and was supportive. She advised us to go to the police. When I saw my daughter in pain, I decided that I had to file a complaint. In all this, my daughter was quiet. We all were supporting her and telling her to tell us the truth about what had happened; we would not say anything to her (we will not blame her or rebuke her). She had already suffered for one and a half months, and we could see from all the marks on her body.

After the examination, we went to the police station to file the rape complaint against the boy. The police started harassing my daughter. One woman constable even slapped her. She said, "You enjoyed all the things at that time, and now you are complaining." She verbally abused her. I told my daughter to ignore it and assured her that I would take it up later. It took us three days to lodge an FIR after the medical examination. When we were at the police station, one senior police officer called me and my husband in the cabin and told us not to file a case. When I asked why, he told me, "If you file a case, then your daughter will be sentenced to seven years of imprisonment." He also said that if we filed a complaint, she would be taken away and kept in a government shelter home as she was a minor. But I decided that I would not bothered about whether or not she was put in the shelter home.

It was not easy for us to file an FIR. I went to Mahila Ayog (State Women's Commission), then to the highest police authority (Police Commissioner's Office) and a human rights organisation. I submitted a letter to each of them stating that I was not getting any justice. My daughter had been missing for one and a half months, and now that she was found, they were not lodging a complaint of rape. So after all this pressure, the police finally took my complaint.

But what they wrote in the complaint is not what we told them. A copy of the FIR was given to me in court, and I was asked to read it and answer the questions according to FIR. But I said, "No, I will not read it out, and I will only tell what I know." In the FIR, the police had mentioned things like my daughter and the boy were in a relationship, they were in love, and both of them were living close by. All this was incorrect, and so I told them that I could not lie.

When my daughter read the FIR, she started arguing in court. She said, "I was there, not you. I was the one who was tied up. I was the one who was crying and not you. I have suffered and not you." She argued with the defence lawyer. She also had marks on her hands and legs as a result of being tied with rope.

The case came up for hearing in court after one year. The accused boy was never brought to the court during case hearings. Whenever I asked about it, they would give some excuse, such as "A vehicle was not available." I wanted to see him, but he was never brought to court. I met his mother in court; even his mother and aunt (Mavshi) were arrested. His mother was released on bail. But his aunt (Mavshi) and that boy were in jail for six months. When Bindu was kidnapped, she was kept in the abuser's aunt's house, and the aunt was aware of what was happening.

The doctor from the public hospital did not come to court. The police called me to ask where I had taken my daughter for medical examination. I told them that I had taken her to that hospital as it is a government hospital. Then the police asked me if I had the address of the doctor who examined Bindu, but I didn't have that. The police said in the court that they looked for the doctor for fifteen days but could not trace her. I don't know what happened, but one month later, they told me that the case was over and he was released. I did not get any paper from the court or police.

I only got a call from the police constable who informed me, "Now don't come to the court as the abuser is released." Then I asked, "How come he is released? I should know the details." So he said, "The court punished him with two years of imprisonment, and as the abuser has already been in jail for that period, he has been released." But I just don't agree with it because he should have been punished for five years as he had harassed and assaulted my child. The police told us that he was released, but according to the lawyers, the boy could not be released like that; he must be out on bail. The boy was twenty-two years old at the time of the incident.

We went to court three to four times, Bindu was called once, and I was called twice. The boy had changed his lawyer seven times. So every time there was a new lawyer, I was called again, and I was asked the same thing again and again. But then I said, "I will not tell you the same thing again and again." During the court hearing, I was also accused of taking money from the accused for withdrawing the case. I told the court that I did not ask for money from the boy or his family and that the money I had received was given to me by the government (Victim Compensation Scheme). I said, "I don't want their money. All I want is to continue with the case and get justice for my daughter." But then the defence lawyer and the boy's family continued to accuse me of filing the case for money. I said, "You can go and ask Mahila Ayog. I got a letter from them stating that they are giving some money for my daughter." We got INR 300,000, and out of which 75,000 was put in a fixed deposit. The defence lawyer's behaviour in court was not right. He was not asking any questions properly; he was threatening us, frightening us, and then posing questions (referring to cross-examination in court). First, he asked me my caste, but then the judge screamed and told him to focus on the case and ask relevant questions. "Don't discuss caste or anything," the judge said to the defence lawyer because there is no relevance of caste in the case. I am a Maharashtrian, but my husband is a Muslim. The defence lawyer then asked me how my marriage was fixed and other things. I said, "Sir, please ask me what is relevant to the case. Please don't ask me about aspects that are not related to the case." Then he asked me, "How did your daughter go with him? When did she go?" I said when she was returning from her class, two people caught her, beat her, and made her drink some yellow-coloured water. All of this has also been mentioned in the medical report. Then he said, "Call your daughter. I will ask her some questions."

So Bindu was also asked by the defence lawyer whether her mother is from another caste (the defence was trying to paint a picture of an unstable family – an inter-religious marriage of parents and a girl having eloped with a boy). She said, "Ask my mother." I know she is from which caste, but if you want this information, then ask her, why ask me? So the defence lawyer was asking the same question again and again by framing it differently. Then he went on to ask, "Where did that boy take you?" He only said one city, so my daughter said loudly, "Please ask me one time only, and I will answer only once." I had told my daughter not to be scared at all, so she was confident in court. I told her that we will lose the case if she will get scared during hearings. The defence lawyer was asking again and again and saying she was taken to two cities. But Bindu was firm on her statement and said, "No, he had taken me to one city." She could remember the dates also, so she told the court, "The boy took me to his auntie's place on this date. I was locked in the room there, was not given food, and was beaten up."

The defence lawyer asked Bindu why she did not scream, so she said, "I was unconscious. How can anyone scream in that condition? If you are tied and made unconscious, will you scream?" Then he said, "That's correct." Bindu said to the defence lawyer, "If you would have been in my place and in that situation, then you would also have spoken loudly in the court. I know what had happened because I have suffered for one and a half months. There was nobody with me, my parents were not there, and they tied me, beat me, and were doing wrong things with me." Then the judge asked everybody to vacate the courtroom and only allowed me, my daughter, and our lawyer to be inside the room. The judge asked all others, including the boy and his relatives, to go out and shut the room, and then the judge asked us to tell everything. Then my daughter was asked about the incident in detail. The public prosecutor used to talk to us properly and used to tell us about the case, but once she asked me to lie in court, which I denied. She gave me some papers to read and took me aside. She asked me to say in court that my daughter was not there for one and a half months and she was pregnant now, but I said I couldn't say so. When she was not pregnant, then how could I say so? Then the lawyer said, "It will make your case strong." I said that the doctor had not told us this, and I could not say so.

She started screaming and said, "Don't you understand? All this has happened with your daughter." I said, "Whatever the situation will be, I cannot lie in court." The medical report was already submitted in the court, so there was no question of telling lies. Being in court was not easy. I was not able to say anything in court. I got scared (*pasine chutate the*) because I had never gone to court before. I shivered in fear when I was giving the statement. The lawyer would hold my hand, and then I talked.

The police used to accompany us to the court and sit with us during the hearing. Also, there were thirty-two witnesses from the abuser's side, and we had no one. The police did not believe us, but the judge believed us. The judge was very good; she said she usually didn't believe in all this (Jadutona), but she trusted us. My daughter told us about one man who had worn lungi and a big Tilak who had come to the locked room. He spread a white sheet, and Bindu was asked to sit on that and drink some water. After drinking that water, he threw lemon and sindur on Bindu's sides, and then he threw some ash (raakh) on her head. There was one transgender person (hijra) also there. Bindu asked them, "What are you doing?" They said, "You just sit. We will get a lot of money." They had cut Bindu's hair and made it short. When I told all this to the judge, she asked the police why they didn't put all this in our complaint. The police said the court would not believe in all this; that's why they didn't record it. To this, the judge said whether the court would believe it or not, the police must mention all this in the complaint. The judge gave the order to arrest everybody who was involved in this case, but the police did not do that. They did not arrest the pandit and hijra; they only arrested the boy, his mother, and his aunt.

My husband and I are daily wage earners. I am a fisherwoman. I go to the dockyard at four in the morning, unload the fish from the boat, and get INR 300 per day. My husband repairs TV and tape, and he does not go out for work because there are children at home. If we both go out, then who will look after the children? I have a daughter who is in twelfth standard now. She is younger than Bindu.

My mother-in-law (MIL) is a homemaker, and my father-in-law (FIL) was in the shipping yard, so he gets a pension. Bindu used to stay with my MIL since her childhood when she was 6 months old. When Bindu went missing, my MIL spent approximately INR 100,000 looking for her. My MIL was so upset that she was not eating food, and her health also got affected.

My daughter suffered a lot. Her treatment was going on for about seven months. She suffered from white discharge also. My MIL took care of the expenses. It cost us INR 50,000–60,000. I have three more children to look after, so MIL's support was necessary.

I did not go back to that public hospital as they were not responding well. When I had taken her, she was screaming in pain, and the staff around kept telling her to stop shouting and wait. When I intervened and told them that she was in acute pain, the nurse told me to leave the room and sit outside. She said, "The girl is just acting up, doing drama." The staff was scolding her, so I did not want to go back there. Then my MIL offered to take care of all expenses related to her treatment. The incident had affected Bindu a lot; she used to behave differently after the incident. She used to tell us to keep the light off, and if we switched it on, she screamed. She was locked in a dark room by the boy. That's why she didn't want the light on (*usko ujala nahi chahiye*) and liked to sit in the dark. She screamed if there was any noise or if anything fell on the ground (any loud sound or sound of breakage). This sound probably reminded her of the violence. Then after six months, I took Bindu to my mother's place, and we stayed there for eight to fifteen days. I took her for outings; everybody took care of her and explained to her that what happened was in the past now and she had a bright future. My other children also were affected. My son was 10 years old, another one was 12, and my daughter was 14 years old. My younger daughter used to say we have not done anything wrong, so we should be strong. Just a few days back, that boy threatened to kill my younger daughter (*tujhe katake rakhunga*). My daughter is brave, and she challenged him to kill her any-time, anywhere! I immediately went to the police station to file a complaint, but the police assured me that they would warn him, and if it ever happens again, then they will take action. She is very smart (*Bohot agau hai*).

Last month, the boy came into our area, and he threatened to kill my younger sister, who was sitting outside. She screamed, and so he ran away. I went to the police station to register a complaint, and they said they would look into it. The boy then called my nephew on the phone and abused him. I again went back to the police and told them that the boy was repeatedly troubling us and pleaded that they take action against him. So police said,

"Your nephew lives on the other side, which is outside our jurisdiction, so go to that police station." Then we went to the other police station. The officer at that police station told us, "As the case is closed, leave it, and if the boy again does anything, then we will see." But I said now it was enough; I am tired of going to the police station.

We were called in at eleven in the morning, and my daughter's statement took two hours. First, his lawyer was asking questions, then our lawyer asked some questions. The judge was checking if there was any difference in the statement that Bindu had given, but she said the same thing each time she was asked. The judge asked what time he used to come in the night, how many times clothes were removed, and how she knew about this. She said, "My hands and legs were tied, but I could feel that my salwar was being removed (*neechese khulla khulla lagta tha*)." She was 16 years old and small, but still, she could understand what was happening.

I could not go to work for three to four months. My mother and sister supported me financially; they took care of our food and looked after my other children. My husband had gone crazy totally (*Puri tarahse pagal hog aye the*); he had lost interest in life. Bindu's condition was like that; anyone who saw her would break down. When my husband gave her tea and bread, she asked him to keep it down on the floor. She refused to eat her food on the plate and licked it from the floor. This is because she was given food on the floor, and she was asked to lick it like a dog. When we were in the police station that time also, she was falling unconscious again and again. If she wanted to go to the toilet, she asked her father to stay near her.

My MIL lives in a building, and there is a toilet inside the house. We went to stay at my MIL's house after Bindu was found. She would keep crying throughout the night. She would keep muttering to herself, saying, "A hijra has come, a burnt woman has come, a pandit has come." She used to demonstrate what those people did to her. We had recorded all her actions on my husband's mobile, but he lost his mobile, and we lost the videos too.

This went on for six to seven months. I used to take her to Dargah, which healed her. One madam had also come to meet her from an organization, but I cannot remember the name. She also told me not to take the case back as Bindu had suffered so much. She said, "Nobody would do this even to an animal. He had harassed and assaulted your daughter brutally." Everybody was telling us not to take tension (not be tensed and worried); they said, "If you take tension, then how will you help your daughter?" We cried continuously, so she asked, "Mummy, why are you crying? I will not die. I will survive." That shook me, and we decided to give it a fight. If we keep crying, then who will take care of her? Everybody in our family was so supportive. I have five SILs (sisters-in-law), five BILs (brothers-in-law), and they were all very supportive. She used to share everything with her grandmother. She said if she liked that boy, then she would have told him so, but the fact is that she did not like him and he had misbehaved with her. There was enmity; he wanted to kill her because she had slapped him. Our neighbours were also supportive. All were helping us to find her.

Bindu had passed her tenth exam and had joined tailoring classes. She wanted to do a course and join the police force. But my MIL was very protective of her and said, "Do whatever you want but at home." My MIL was scared and so was not in favour of her joining the police. Bindu would say, "I will become police and will punish them."

My MIL later vacated that room and shifted to another area. She took my daughter with her saying it would help her to forget what had happened. So as soon as the case was closed, they shifted there. Bindu started taking care of the children from the neighbourhood. There was one clinic near the house, and the doctor at the clinic suggested that he would teach Bindu small things about nursing, such as giving an injection. Thus, Bindu went to work at the clinic.

I don't want to do anything further now because Bindu is happily married. But I would like to know why and how he was acquitted – whether they bribed or if they did anything because his mother was very cunning (*chalakh thi*) and politically connected.

It is my MIL who got Bindu back to life and helped her forget all the bad memories. Later, there was a marriage proposal from her present husband, and we decided to get her married. She is happy, and everything is going on well. I told her about our meeting, so she said she would also like to come.

6   Woh ("If he is innocent then am I the criminal?") – Rani

Rani was 17 years old when she was kidnapped by a young man and his friends who lived in her neighbourhood. The man had been following her to college and harassing her. Four men kidnapped her and took her to a place in Mumbai where she was kept for two days and then was taken to another state where she was kept for three months till she was rescued. Her parents had a tough time registering a police complaint, and it was recorded as a missing case only after intervention from senior officials and a minister. The incident occurred in September 2013, when she was drugged and was repeatedly subjected to violence and rape. A medical examination took place in December 2013. A surgical abortion was provided when Rani was found to be five and a half weeks pregnant. The products of conception (POC) were taken for DNA analysis. The harassment by the accused and his aides continued, and a number of complaints have been filed since April 2014. The family faced a lot of harassment from the abuser's families and neighbourhood. Several complaints were registered, but the police did not take action. The court hearing started at the end of January 2015 and repeated applications to court for cancellation of bail of accused were rejected. We met Rani soon after the court acquitted the accused.

Interview with Rani conducted three years after the incident

I was kidnapped/abducted by four people. They forced me to take some pills, and then I had no idea what had happened. The men who kidnapped me were living in our neighbourhood. The father of the main accused works in a bar. His mother used to work earlier, but now she doesn't work. They are rich people. The boy used to work somewhere, but now he builds houses.

When the first time my mother went to file a police complaint, one policeman threatened her, saying, "If you file a case, there is a lot of procedure involved and no one will believe you." Soon, other policemen also started saying the same thing. The first response of the police was bad. They did not

DOI: 10.4324/9781003281887-7

listen to me at all and beat me up. They also beat my father. My mother went to several police stations in our area and also met the minister. The police were not listening to us as the accused had bribed them. We met a local elected representative also. My mother also went to Mantralaya. But no one heard us out. They all abused us and used very foul language (she broke down). Those from the accused side even threatened to kill me, but every time we tried to register a complaint, the police demanded a bribe. Wherever we went, the accused and his aides followed us there. They mocked us, saying no one will believe us. Later, when the minister gave us a letter, then the police heard us out. This was when my parents went to file a police complaint when I did not return home. They called the accused and questioned them about the place where I had been locked up. The police demanded money from my parents to bring me back from there. My parents had to take a loan to give this money (bribe) to the police. Only after the money was paid to the police did they go to that city (in another state of India). They arrested only three of them and left the fourth one. To date, they have not arrested the fourth person or brought him to court as he is a rich person.

The police filed a missing complaint on their own. My mother never said that I had gone missing. Her complaint was for kidnapping. She went to three police stations. They made my mother run here and there till 1:00 a.m. At 1:00 a.m. they filed her complaint. When my father came to the police station at 11:00 p.m., the police rudely told him to go away. The police had to be reminded that they had only insisted on the presence of my father in the police station for registering a complaint. The police kept saying to my parents, "Your daughter has married the boy, so she will not come now." The boy's family threatened to beat up my family. The boy's father openly proclaimed that his son had taken me (their daughter) and my family couldn't do anything about it. He openly challenged my parents to go wherever they wished to any police station or any other place, saying that they could cause him no harm at all (*mera kuch nahi ukhdega).* He said he had already paid INR 50,000 to the police, so that was the reason no one was listening to their complaint. It was only when my family sought support from politicians our plea was heard. In the third month after my disappearance, an FIR was filed. The entire system abused us a lot. The police brought me back from the eastern state after three months. After they brought me back to Mumbai, they put me and that boy in the same room in police custody. Nobody was present in the room, not even the police. He had abused me a lot. He had beaten me with a pipe and verbally abused me. I was 17 years old, and he was 30.

The police were not listening to anything and were saying that it was my fault. They wanted us to give a statement in favour of the boy, which we refused. They beat up my father and my uncle and tried to beat up my mother also in front of the boy's parents. But I said I would not do that. Why would I say anything in favour of him? They are all "big" people in our locality. That's why all this pressure was put on us. They just wanted us to say that I went on my own with him.

When they came to hit my mother, she said, "See, don't touch me. You are not touching his parents, and then why are you touching me? I am from the girl's side, but now if you will touch, then I won't leave you. We have tolerated a lot of abuses from you, but now I won't tolerate this." My mother has been running around so much in the last three years. She went to every place and every politician (*neta*).

After a lot of abuse, the police filed the complaint. We were made to sit, and the officer kept typing on the computer and then took my mother's thumbprint on a paper. We don't know whether the information written in our complaint was right or wrong. We said we wanted to read what was written. They refused and then took us to the municipal hospital. They did not give us a copy of the FIR. They made my mother write a letter that Rani went on her own with the boy. We were at the police station from 10:00 a.m. The whole day they kept us in the police station, from morning till night. Then we didn't know from where they called a lawyer. The lawyer told us not to file the case. He said, "You will suffer a lot, so don't do it."

At the municipal hospital, everything was fine. They kept me for two days. I was pregnant for over one month, and I wanted an abortion. Everyone behaved well in the municipal hospital, and we met one social worker also. The police came to the hospital and took my signature on some paper. In the hospital too, they took my signature before the examination. He had given me pills and beaten me with a pipe. We told the police and also the hospital. But they said the marks are quite old. I still suffer from the pain.

After discharge from the hospital, the police called us to the police station. I was not able to walk properly at that time and used to faint sometimes. They called that day at 9:00 p.m. I said that I could not come, but they insisted, so I went there with my mother and aunt. The lawyer was present too in the police station. The boys were arrested after eight days. The police had taken lots of money as a bribe from the accused. So the pleas of only the accused were heard. Our plea was not heard anywhere.

When the court case started, the abuser started abusing me and said that he had won. He said he would not leave me and my family if he was punished. Even if he would be sentenced for two years, he said he would come out and teach us a lesson. I have the recording of all that he said. I did not have a mobile phone at that time. An acquaintance later gave one to my father.

The abusers were out on bail very soon, within a few days, and kept abusing my family members. They kept pressuring us to withdraw the case and would threaten us all the time. They have been threatening us throughout. After the court granted them bail, they distributed sweets to everyone in our neighbourhood as if they had won the case. They submitted a bond of INR 70,000 or more. I don't know the exact amount. They were even given a restraining order (tadipar) to not enter our area.

The previous public prosecutor was very good, and he was very supportive. But the current one is not supportive; he doesn't know anything about us. The previous lawyer used to counter the defence lawyer in court, but the present lawyer does not say anything. The earlier one who represented the case for six months always used to come to court on time, but this one does not. He had managed to get the bail order cancelled, but he soon retired. The accused was not arrested again (the order for bail cancellation was not implemented). The public prosecutor never met us. Even when *didi* (counsellor) tried to meet her, she avoided us, saying she would talk later. So we never knew the status of the case.

The abusers tried various tactics to prevent us from pursuing the case in court. They assaulted my mama (maternal uncle) when the case was going on. He suffered fractures to his hands and legs and other severe injuries to his ears.

All the people in the neighbourhood are scared of them. They are goons. There is one person from the neighbourhood who took signatures of people from our area against us. He got everyone to sign a paper to say that everyone in the neighbourhood was on the boy's side.

People around us told us that they were willing to sign a statement in support of us also. My mother asked them, "What sense does it make to support both parties?" They were not present there, so what do they know? I told them, "I am the one who was abused, and only I know what happened to me."

This man from the neighbourhood was paid INR 20,000 by that boy to take all these signatures. After this, the local politician called for a meeting of about two hundred people. They asked my mother to be present and told her to come alone for a meeting without my father. They wanted to threaten my mother in front of everyone. They even offered money to her. What was my mother going to do in front of two hundred people? So she did not go to that meeting. They came to our house at 1:00 a.m. and abused us and questioned us for not coming for the meeting. These people were from our neighbourhood as well as from outside. They kept taunting my mother for not going to that meeting. They would pass comments, such as "She has become very big (meaning a strong person not afraid of the threats), so does not listen to us."

Their main agenda was to ensure that my parents should withdraw the complaint and get me married to that boy. Why would we not pursue the case? I knew what I had been through, so I would fight the case. I was determined to not let them off – come what may. And mind you, it was not a marriage proposal from the accused, but they just wanted us to say this before the court.

One of the abusers said he would take me from there, and another one threatened to kill us. He said he would cut us to pieces. He openly offered INR 100,000 to anyone willing to kill us. We came to know this through a person from our village who overheard all this.

Our lives have changed completely since the incident. The abusers harass us all the time. My mother accompanies my siblings to school as she is afraid that the abusers will cause harm. My brother keeps telling my mother not to come to school, but she is scared. The accused is always with a group of people, moving around freely, spending money on others, and has everyone's support.

Whenever a new person comes into the neighbourhood, abusers show them my photo and tell them everything about me. They show them my nude photographs that they had taken. So all the time, they are trying to defame me everywhere (*niche girana chahte hai*). We have complained about this to the police and also to the court. But no action was taken. The computer was also not seized by the police.

We don't socialise with anyone now. I keep the door of our house closed all the time. There have been fights over water from the public tap in the past, so we don't interact much. In one such incident, the abusers had threatened me that they would teach me a lesson in one or two months. The abusers would start a fight whenever I stepped out of the house. I used to answer back, but they were abusive. They keep talking bad things about me. They say that I lived with him for three months and became pregnant. (She started crying.)

I was good at my studies, but I had to stop going to college. They would follow me when I went to college. So now I just stay at home. My elder sister continued her college, but she failed because of all this, and now she is also at home. My brothers are going to school. I want to study, but they still harass me. Wherever I go, they follow me. I have been in the house for the last four years and go out only with my mother.

People keep telling my parents to marry me to someone or send me to the village. The house we live in was bought by my father a few years back. He sells jalebis (an Indian sweet that is freshly fried and sold on carts). We already have a loan of more than a lakh.

Not only are these boys all goons, their uncle, too, is in jail for killing someone. We all want to see them punished for what they did to me, and I want them to be in jail for at least ten years.

My paternal uncle fears that they will harm his children, so he doesn't support us. But my maternal uncle is supportive. We have no other support, and there is pressure from everyone to withdraw the case. People say that my mother is brave and courageous to have taken up this fight (for justice). She is hopeful that our plea will be heard one day. She says that even if she dies, she has four children who will fight the case, and someday there will be justice. People around us left no opportunity to discourage us. (She started crying.) But whenever this *didi* (counsellor) comes, she tells us not to lose courage.

That's where I got the courage. Otherwise, everyone from the neighbourhood had discouraged me (*mujhe niche gira diya tha*), be it *bhaiyya* (migrants) or *Marathi* (locals) – everyone discouraged me. I used to help the neighbours with many things like children's projects or *mehndi*. But now, I don't do it as they taunt me after their work is done. So when they approach me now, I say, "I am *chinar* (adultress). I am *randi* (prostitute), right? That's what you call me? I will not do this for you."

People abuse me a lot. My mother is fostering the son of my uncle as my aunt is dead. He goes to the municipality school. When my mother goes to pick him from the school in the afternoon, they pass all kinds of comments: "See, she is going to get herself fucked (*gand marane ja rahi hai)*"

My father is the only earning member. For three months, when we were trying to file a complaint, his business was closed. We had to borrow INR 30,000 for household expenses. Throughout the case, we had to go to court twice a month. So his work also got affected. And then the municipality will sometimes allow to put up the food stall and will not allow other times. There is a problem with everything. If they take away the stall, then they have to be paid INR 3,000–5,000. He has to pay the bribe (*hafta)* of INR 50 per day for putting his stall.

Now whenever my mother steps out of the house, my elder sister starts crying. After the last episode, my sister does not allow my mother to step outside the house. (She started to cry.) She says, "You are going alone. Somebody will kill you. Then who will be there for us? If they kill you on the road, then what will we do? Who will be there for us?"

I live with this fear every day. We are always worried. Whenever our mother steps out, we say, "Mummy, come home fast, be careful while going. Otherwise, someone will kill you." The school is a bit far away. They have to walk as we cannot afford the auto fare. We don't have a TV – we keep asking for it, but my father already has a lot of debt. He says it will take two years at least to clear our debt. People say that we are fighting a false case. I will fight, come what may.

The police said, "We are policemen, and so you should be afraid of us, and take your case back." But I said I wouldn't take the case back even if I am killed. My mother said, "Someone in this world will listen to our complaints." People keep coming home to pressure us to "compromise" (settle the case out of court). My mother tells them to leave, saying it is none of their concern. "They gave you money. Go to them, do not come to me. If you come again, I will go to the police station." So they just threaten us and leave. They even say that I am ready to get married to the abuser, but my mother is not letting me do it. All these talks happen behind our backs. One day I was going to school to get my result sheet (report card), when a boy spat on me. I retaliated by shouting at him. Now, whenever they see me, they spit because they have won the case.

We are not very old in the area where we are living presently. We have already bought a house here and now what to do? We can't go back to our old locality. The rent is INR 10,000–12,000 over there. How can we afford it? If we pay that much rent, what will we eat?

All we want is that he should be punished for what he has done. Other people in the neighbourhood say terrible things about me.

7 "We were forced to leave the city due to continued abuse. Is this fair on my kids?" – Anu

Timeline

Anu, 25 years of age, came to the hospital at 12:30 p.m. in August 2014 and was examined at 2:15 p.m. She was brought by the police. The incident had occurred in December 2013 and was repeated several times. The abuser had a video of Anu and her daughter in the nude and threatened to make it public. He continued to rape her. Later, he asked for her gold earrings and demanded money. It was only then that Anu gathered up the courage to tell her husband. A case of rape was registered, but the abuser was granted bail within three months on the condition that he would not live in the same area. But he continued to live there and threatened Anu and her family routinely. The court case is moving slowly. She had filed several complaints against him, but the police have not taken any action.

Interview with Anu three years after the incident

He (the abuser) is unmarried and lives in our neighbourhood only. He has two sisters and parents. Both his sisters are married, but they stay in our area only. My in-laws knew his family for several years and had very good relations with them. They were so close that whenever my in-laws would go out of town, they would give their keys to the abuser's family members. We had a tortoise at home that had to be given water and looked after, so his parents would do all that. But after the incident, everything changed. The abuser distributes newspapers (*paper dalata hai*) and goes house to house. He is not a politician or anything, but still no one says anything to him. I don't know why.

He was troubling me a lot (*yane uska na bohot jadahi ho gaya tha*) and had started demanding money and my jewellery. I thought a lot about it at that time, and then I finally told everything to my husband. My husband said we would file a complaint against the abuser. We went to the police station and told them what had happened and sought their advice on what should

DOI: 10.4324/9781003281887-8

be done. So when we met the senior officer over there, he suggested that we should file an FIR against the abuser. They took my statement, and it got over at 10:00–10:30 p.m. Then the police went to arrest the abuser (*apradhi*). They (police) arrested him immediately and brought him to the police station. I had reached the police station at 3:30 p.m. and came back home at 1:30 a.m. The police wanted to take me at night for a medical examination, but my husband said it was too late, so we went the next day.

At the hospital, the doctor asked me what had happened. So I told them everything – all that had happened to me. The doctor behaved properly with me. I was not kept waiting there. There was one lady doctor who checked me. Whatever she asked me, I answered her. We had gone for medical at around 10:00–10:30 a.m., and we came back home at around 3:00–3:30 p.m.

This was the first time we had filed an FIR against the abuser. The abuser was arrested. He was in jail for about three to three and a half months.

After he came out on bail, he and his family members tortured us a lot. The abuser used to follow me when I used to go out to drop my children at school. He used to stand in my way, hold my hand, and touch me all over my body. He would do this repeatedly. We have complained to the police several times. I also called the police helpline 100 every time he harassed me. The police would hear me out, note something, and even call him to the police station, but before I reached home, he would be set free. This has happened so many times. The police made us sit in the police station till 11:00 p.m. just to file a non-cognisable complaint (NC).

The police never asked me any awkward questions. They wrote down exactly what I told them. But they used to write very basic and simple (non-cognisable) complaints (*aikdum sadhi complaint likhate hai who log*). The police would call the abuser and his aides (*dalal log*) to the police station, but every time, they managed to leave immediately. After the first FIR, not once was the abuser arrested for his continued harassment and threats.

I will tell you what happened after a recent incident of harassment by the abuser. That day I was on my way to pick up my daughter from school. So I picked her up and went to the police station to file a complaint. I told them that the abuser followed me to school and caught my hand. I reminded the police officer that last time when I came to report this matter, he suggested that I should call the 100 police helpline number and assured me that he would not get away like this. I told him, "Therefore, I have come to you with my daughter straight from school." They asked me to wait, and I was there till 8:00 p.m., and they had not taken my complaint. I called my husband from the police station only and told him everything and asked him to come there. My husband immediately came there to the police station.

My husband then asked me what happened. I told him everything. Then my husband questioned the police regarding this, so they told my husband that policemen had gone to arrest the abuser. They even asked my husband to accompany them so that the abuser could be identified. My husband went along with them; he took our daughter with him as she was hungry and had been waiting at the police station for a very long time after school. I sat in the police station. The police brought one man, but he was the abuser's brother (*mausi ka ladka*). I told the police that he was not the one (abuser), so the police hit the abuser's brother a lot, saying, "Why did you lie?" After ten to fifteen minutes, the abuser came to the police station. Police kept him seated and took my statement. I was asked what happened, so I narrated how he followed me and harassed me and how I was forced to take an auto as my daughter was waiting alone in school due to all the delay caused by him. I told them he followed me everywhere. He held my hand and touched my breasts from behind and did all other things, and therefore, I had come to make a complaint. So the police made a note and called him. I was asked to wait. Then his family member came, and along with them, there was one Dalal (someone who settled matters by offering bribes). I think that Dalal used to work in the police station. He was an ex-policeman and had some conversation with the police, and they let the abuser go. Per the bail order, he was told not to step into our area. But he had given the address of his sister's marital home in Worli as his current residence to the police and court. When his sister is living here, how is it possible for the abuser to be living with his sister's in-laws? We provided all these facts to the police, but they accepted his version. He had been telling the police he came here only to meet his parents as they were not in good health. He was also carrying on with his paid work here.

My experience with the police had been very difficult. I would like to say that if anybody (emphatically) goes to make a police complaint, then that person should get help (*Uski madat karni chahiye*). The person should not be told, "Yes, I will do it, you sit." All this should not be happening. The person should be treated properly. Many times when anyone goes to file a complaint, then they are just asked to wait for hours. The police keep doing their other work, and we remain seated there, waiting. When we sit there, everybody keeps looking at you, which makes us feel very bad and dirty (*ganda lagta hai*) (emphatic while saying this).

Now I don't stay in the area and come only when there is a court hearing and leave immediately after the hearing for my children.

We decided to shift to another state because of continuous threats from abuser. He threatened to kill my children (*bacche log ko mar dalunga)* and defame my family (*tere parivar ki badnami karunga*). I was scared about his threats to harm my children. If anything happens to my children, then there is just nothing left for me. I will lose everything (*mera toh gaya hi na fir*).

My children will have to be dropped at school every day, and if he does anything like that, each time my husband had to come from work and had to take leave. My husband's office had issued memos twice for taking too many leaves from work.

After the incident, even people in the neighbourhood started behaving badly with us. Everybody in the neighbourhood was on his side, and nobody was on our side. Whenever I used to pass by, the people in the neighbourhood used to talk something behind me. This has affected us all. My daughter was 4–5 years old at that time, but nobody allowed her to play with their children. They told their children not to play with my daughter, so my daughter cried a lot at home. Whenever this topic comes up, my daughter just clamps up. She is eleven years old now and understands it a little bit, so she suddenly becomes silent (*ekdum sunn ho jati hai who*). My younger child was just 2 years old at that time; therefore, he does not know about it.

Over the years, some people around us have now begun to communicate with us. But nobody talks about the case. This boy had done the same thing with three to four women, but only I had taken action against him, and therefore, I became bad in everybody's eyes (*Sabke aankh me aa gayi*).

My husband is very supportive and comes with me for every court hearing. My marital family knows about it, but I have not told my natal family. They live in another state. I have two sisters-in-law (SILs) and two brothers-in-law (brother-in-law), and they also know about it and support me as well. My father-in-law (FIL) is with us, but he is old, and it is difficult for him to climb the stairs here (in Mumbai). So whenever I have to come here for the court case, he looks after both my children. We have not got any summons yet, but we have gathered information from the internet. (She showed some papers.)

I had gone to court three to four times. Once, the female judge had asked me directly, "What problem do you have? He says he is living in Worli." So I told her that the Worli address is that of his sister's marital home, but his sister stays with her parents in our area. I asked the judge, "Do you think his sister-in-law will allow him to stay there?" I told her that I had informed all this to the police also, but no action had been taken.

The abuser's lawyer informed in the court that the abuser has filed cases (false allegations) against me and my husband, but we were not aware of it until then. There was a cross NC against us, and only in the court did we come to know about it.

So now the next hearing is in February, and I don't know what will happen. There was a case hearing in January also, but that day, nothing happened. The abuser's lawyer had not come that day. We had submitted an application for cancellation of the abuser's bail, but the application was not accepted. We are planning to submit it again. The application was not accepted, as I did not have any identity proof at that time. Now I have my documents, and I will submit the application once again. People should get justice, madam. It's been so many years of my case. I should not have had to face the difficulties that I am facing right now. If he had been punished soon, then I would have continued to live in Mumbai, which would not have affected my children's studies.

Whenever there is a date in the court, I have to leave my children with someone for dropping and picking them from school. Every time I have to depend on someone. My elder daughter understands because she knows how rape cases are dealt with. She has seen similar cases on TV shows, so she understands, and when I come here, I tell her that I am going for the case. I tell her that I will be away for the entire day so stay carefully at home for a day with your grandfather.

I get very angry (was crying) when I think about all this. Therefore, I have made my mind that now I will not leave him and he should be punished. I will do whatever I would have to do. I just think that I have to fight and should get justice. My husband also tells me the same thing: "So much has happened. You have borne so much. Now just stay strong and lift your spirit."

We have spent a lot of money on the case. I have a public prosecutor, so we don't have to give anything to him, but lots of money go into travelling. Each trip costs INR 300 from home to court. I spend a minimum of INR 1,000 during one court hearing. The shifting (relocation) from one city to another has affected my children's studies a lot (negative impact). There is a huge difference between (quality of) education here and what is available there. Both my children have become dull. My elder daughter was very sharp and used to talk promptly and write a lot. Her father says she will take some time to adjust because it's a new school. She will make new friends there also, and children these days do harass newcomers.

Due to this, my daughter gets upset. She says, "Mamma, I do not want to stay here. I don't like this school." She tells my husband to stay with mummy and brother, and she will go back and live with her grandmother. (She laughed nervously.) So her father explains to her that we have to adjust. Now she has her final exam next month because it is the central board. There was a change from the state board to the central board. The syllabus was heavy for her, and she had to cover up a lot in a short time. I also want to come back here, but who will ensure the safety of me and my family?

8 "They have mentioned on record that physical and mental cruelty by the husband has happened, but no mention of sexual cruelty." – Neeta

Neeta, 38 years old, was brought by police to the hospital in June 2014 at 12:43 p.m. She had been subjected to forced sexual intercourse, including oral penetration by the husband, for several years but had filed a complaint of marital rape only after twenty years of marriage.

Interview with Neeta three years after she filed the complaint

It was in December, 2010. We had gone to a place close by for an outing with his (husband's) friends, the two of us, and our kids. As it was New Year's Eve, the men in the group had a drinking party (had a few drinks). His friend's wife and I were busy the whole day cooking, washing utensils, and serving the men and kids whatever they wanted. We were doing it, happily thinking that it was a family party. At night, as we were very tired, we went to sleep at around 10:30–11:00 p.m. There was no maid for any of the domestic work over there, so it was very tiring. In a few seconds, I was fast asleep. I was sleeping next to my son. My husband's friend's son, who was fifteen years old, came and slept next to my son at some point in the night. I don't know when he came and slept there. Around 2:30–3:00 a.m., my husband came into the room. He kicked me in my lower back, and it was so hard that it hurt me badly, and so I screamed in pain. I was sleeping on the floor on a mattress as there were no cots over there. When I opened my eyes and looked up at him, he was constantly kicking me. I was not able to understand what was happening.

As I was screaming with pain, all others came running to our room. My husband told them to leave the room. I was lying on the floor and could not get up due to pain. I was crying, so my husband told everyone, "She is "psychic" (someone who has a mental health disorder) and she always screams at night." He said that I had a psychological problem and how this caused a lot of trouble and embarrassment in society as everyone kept asking him

DOI: 10.4324/9781003281887-9

about what happened. I was devastated when I heard this. First of all, I was not screaming without reason. I was screaming because I was beaten up by him, and he had kicked me with his shoes.

I was wondering, where did I go wrong? I slept just as everyone else decided to. I kept on thinking for the whole night and trying to find the reason why he hit me. I could not find any reason, but in the morning, when I kept asking him for the reason, I came to know that he could not have sex with me as there was the other boy in the room, and so in the fit of anger, he did all this. After returning from the trip, I narrated the entire incident to my daughter, who was 16 years old then. My daughter confronted her father.

She questioned him for beating me in front of outsiders and calling me a psychic. He retorted, "Is your mother not ashamed of herself for sleeping next to that 15-year-old boy?" My daughter said, "What is there to be ashamed about? The boy is even younger than me, and there is nothing wrong that she has done." Then I decided enough was enough now. Now if he made any demand for sex, I decided not to respond, and then I completely stopped giving in to his demands for sex. This was in January 2011.

He used to demand oral sex also. Initially, he used to beg in front of me for oral sex and would promise to do whatever, like getting groceries, looking after me, and so on. He would plead in front of me. He would be a different person when asking for oral sex but never fulfilled anything that he promised to do later. But till the time I did not do whatever he was asking for, he would not leave me. He used to keep following me at home wherever I went. I used to fear that kids may wake up and would come to know everything. So I used to think that if I did it now, then all this would end in fifteen minutes to half an hour, and then I could at least sleep and he would be satisfied (*shant hoil*), and then I used to give in to his demands.

This demand for oral sex started after a few years of marriage. We got married in 1994, so till 2000, there was no such demand. It all started after that. He started making all kinds of demands and would warn me that if I didn't do it, he could go out and buy it for INR 200–500 (buy sex). This went on from 2000 to 2010. Many times I felt like sharing this with my friends. I have two very close friends at the school where I teach, and both of them are older than me. I even thought of sharing with them by telling them that this is happening with a friend of mine. But I was not able to share it with anyone. I was not aware that such things happen, and this is also one type of sex. Afterwards, when I started reading about it, I realised that these can be with mutual consent too. Many times both partners like it, or if one partner likes it, then the other partner convinces her/him. But my husband never discussed it with me or tried to understand what I felt or what I desired or never took medical help.

I used to say many times to him, "You like it, but I don't, so let us once discuss with a doctor why I don't like it. And what should I do to enjoy it."

He also used to say, "You don't give me this, you don't give me that. All the household comforts are for you. None of the comforts are for me. This AC is for you, this big house is for you, none of this is for me." So I used to wonder, both of us are staying in this house, whatever amenities there are, are for both of us, and they are equal. How come they are only for me?

In 2009, I changed my doctor, Dr B, a homoeopathic physician. Later he became our family doctor also. During the first visit, the doctor notes down the history of the patient in detail, including life history. The doctor told me to take some time and write down the detailed history at home and also gave me a form that had many columns about marital life, my children, aspirations, and overall attitude towards life. So I had written a little bit about the abuse from my husband in that form. Then when he was talking with me, he had asked me about it. I was able to tell him about it. So I could disclose it only then.

The doctor was the first person I spoke to. He was a male doctor, but he approached it in a very friendly manner, and he told me, "If you don't like it (oral sex), you have the right to say no." So that was the first time I realised that I can say no to him. But I was not able to say no, and even if I said no, he did not listen to it and forced me to do it.

But then that incident happened. My daughter was the first one to see it. My husband forced oral penetration on my son. I started blaming myself for having stayed in this house for so many years. I suffered for so many years, and then my son had to go through the same thing. It was not my son's responsibility to provide him (husband) sex. This was not acceptable, and I kept thinking about how this 6-year-old boy (son) may have felt. I am so troubled because of it and never got any satisfaction from it (in tears), so what did he (son) feel? And I also thought that he might grow up and develop hatred for all these things (sex). What would he do? I was not able to understand anything. And I said to him, "Son, why didn't you tell me?" I asked him this as he told us that this had happened several times. My daughter and I both asked him why he didn't tell us. "Had you told us, we would have ensured that this did not happen to you." So he promptly and angrily said to me, "You could not save yourself. How would you have saved me?" When I heard him, that moment I realised that according to him, I was very weak and unable to defend myself. I get beaten up (*mar khanari ahe*), and he was right, how could he have complained to me? He believed that his mother could not have helped him as she was unable to save herself. So then I decided that I needed to become strong. He should feel that his mother was strong, she was a fighter, and she could fight, which meant he should have that confidence. I should make him capable and provide him with that security that whatever happened had happened, but in the future, he should speak up and defend himself. If someone was doing such an act against our will, we should be able to speak up and stand against it. He must be assured that his mother was becoming strong or rather that she was strong.

At that moment, I decided that I could not continue in this house any longer. I called my natal family and informed them about what had happened. My father believed that it must be some misunderstanding: maybe it was just his imagination (*bhram zala asel*), my husband must not be having such intentions, he must have touched my son's private parts while bathing him, my son may have perceived it wrongly, and so on. But my mother strongly supported me and said, "You are feeling this, then I will support you. You just think about it calmly and take a decision based on what you feel is right. You have my firm support."

At that time, I told everything to my mother because I felt confident that she was with me. I was working at the school all this while. I have friends who work in an NGO, they are A D and P Y. I discussed everything with them because at that time, I was working with them on a research study called "Facebook and Friendship." I told them what had happened in my house and that I might not be able to continue working. Both of them came to my natal home, spoke with me, and provided a lot of support. They spoke with my daughter as well. I was feeling that my daughter did not know much about our personal life, but unfortunately (to my surprise), she knew everything. She was aware that I used to cry at night, that he (husband) used to take me from the bedroom to hall or kitchen; she knew everything. My daughter said that she was not able to sleep for many nights. My friend said that I could seek justice by filing a case of domestic violence. They informed me about a women cell in the police station. They told me to go there and file a domestic violence case and a separate case for my son. My friends also called my husband there and observed his attitude in the way he spoke and behaved while he was there. After seeing all that, they said, "You will require legal help. It does not seem like the matter can be settled out of court through mutual understanding." They advised me to go to court and file a divorce case before my husband filed a case against me with various allegations. They also said that I could be questioned for not doing anything when my son was sexually abused. Any woman would ask for a divorce in such circumstances as she would not want to keep any relation with such a man.

My friend was a great support to me, and she even became a witness in court. She reminded me about an incident during a pilgrimage that we had travelled together. I bought some guavas. I like hard, unripe guavas, so I bought those. My husband had not told me about the type of guava I should bring for him. So I bought one kilogram of hard guavas, and he had thrown hard guava at my forehead. It had hit me so badly that I still have a bump on my forehead. He hit me in front of everyone who was there on the bus with us. At that time, many people on the bus asked me why I was putting up with this man and his behaviour. He could not even control his anger or just exchange the guavas if he did not like them. For such a trivial reason, beating was not right. Even the people on the bus were feeling sorry and knew what was happening was very wrong.

My world at that time was also not that big. It was centred around school, home, and kids. So because of that, I was not aware of how other women's husbands behaved. I don't know. Maybe at that time, my thinking was not broad. I went through all this for 17 years. I collapsed in 2012. I took treatment as I was suffering from depression.

All my symptoms were of depression. I would carry out activities on the advice of my lawyers, but later one day, I was simply unable to recall anything. I was worried – what if someone had taken advantage of me or I had fallen off the train? I was taking medicines at the time for dealing with depression, which would make my head heavy. When I told this to my doctors, they reduced the medicines. Later a friend told me that one of those days when I met her, my hair were messed up. I had given her a leave application to be given to school, but she later told me that I had just scribbled on that paper. I had scribbled in the place of signature too. I still have that piece of paper in my file.

Now, I have become very strong, which means now if he throws one guava at me, I will throw back one hundred guavas at him. I have become strong because of my friends in the NGO, my mother, and my children – my daughter also stood by me. I would keep searching about the issue on the internet and social media platforms. Many people guided me whenever I called them for support. All of this helped me to become strong. In the past, whenever someone said something to me, I used to cry a lot. So probably that was a symptom of depression. If anyone said anything to me, I would cry. For example, the principal (where she works) may scold me and others, but I was the one who would cry a lot. I just could not bear it, but now when he (principal) said anything, I couldn't tolerate it. I stopped him and explained the situation. I told him that he had misunderstood and if he wanted this work done urgently, we would submit it within half an hour.

My colleagues supported me a lot. Once, my colleague who is retired now intervened on my behalf in a meeting with the principal. My colleague said, "Are you aware of the kind of harassment she is suffering? She is suffering from physical harassment, sexual harassment." So I just held her hand and tried to tell her not to speak about it, but she said, "Let me tell them, and make them understand." At that time, everyone had become still and were listening, but nobody came to me, held me, or consoled me. No one said, "Don't cry, we are there with you," but they all praise me now as I have become confident. I am not in contact with marital family, and they do not have any role to play in this entire matter. Running the house on my own was a challenge. In the past, my passbook, cheque, PAN card, and all the policy documents, even my jewelry, were with my husband. So when I had to wear jewelry for any function, he gave it to me. I was allowed to wear it only for that much time. Once we returned home, I had to give it back to him. I did not have any financial freedom. The fact is that after I stepped out of the house, I could at least spend the money on my terms. I also came to realise that he had spent all my money and he had it all planned.

That is what I feel. When I stepped out of the house, I only had INR 1,400, and he had around 20–25 lakh in his bank account. I guess he did all this so that I could never think of stepping out of the house. The counsellor had told me that many men keep control over their wives. They fear that if the woman is financially strong, then she will be able to walk out of the house, so they make her weak.

So this happened to me also. I had no bank balance and had to entirely depend on my father. Initially, my father gave me INR 40,000. I said I wanted to at least buy a fridge and washing machine. I bought these two things by taking money from my father. I stayed with my parents for three months and later we started staying on rent near my school. I have now bought my own house – a one-room kitchen.

I will tell you about my experience with the police and court. I think police do not want to understand or they do not understand, which means what we are telling does not reach their brain, or maybe they understand but show as if they do not understand. They make such mistakes that the woman only has to bear the effects of those mistakes. Like I mentioned, all my valuables were in the locker, and only my husband had access to those. So when my husband was in prison for seventeen days, the police should have checked the locker. But they did not do that. They did it after one and a half months of my husband's release from jail. So he had adequate time to take out the things from the locker.

It could have been proven in court that he had operated the locker, but when we asked for CCTV footage, the bank said that the files were corrupted. But the police did not try to recover that footage by taking the hard disk and sending it to the forensic department. All of this was possible to do. I have read a lot about this, and so I am saying this. But the police have no will to do anything. These are all trivial matters for them, according to police, and for them, only murders or other bigger crimes are important.

They feel that crimes against women are trivial (*phutkal vattat*) because they look at it only as a husband-wife quarrel, and they keep on mentioning, "He is your husband after all," and they constantly suggest a settlement. But what are your offerings to me in that settlement? Settlements for the sake of settlement. Judges, too, want women to settle the cases and not pursue it (seek justice).

Judges don't use their authority anywhere. It's not like they are saying, "Okay, I will do a settlement for you, so you offer this much alimony to the woman. Or if you are offering this much, then I will go ahead with the procedure." I mean, I just don't understand whether they don't understand or their attitude is that way or whether their upbringing has happened that way or they are also a part of our society, so even they feel that a settlement is right. I observed this in the high court, and it is written on their faces: "the woman is lying" (*Bai khota bolte*). Something of this sort is always seen on their faces. So they believe that women are lying and, therefore, are biased about it. When it comes to court, I feel the level to which they should have interrogated they did not. They didn't take the case to the extent to which they should have taken. This is what I feel. My public prosecutor had told me, "You have written down your complaints so well, in detail, but you should have mentioned the abusive words that he used." She said when such cases come up for hearing, merely saying in court "he abused me" is not enough. It is important to mention the exact words. In the same way, even the police should have asked what happened and on what date it happened. Or even in the case of my son, he should not have been taken to the police station. There is a legal provision that instructs the police that they should meet children at a place where he is comfortable. But that did not happen with my son.

Also when I took my son to the doctor at the government hospital, the police asked us to travel by train. It was mentioned in my son's statement itself, "I am afraid of trains because my father used to say that he will throw me in front of a train if I tell my mother," so this is so important. In his one-page statement, the child is saying that he is afraid of a particular thing, yet they are asking us to travel by the same mode of transport. Police should have some sense. I said that I would spend money and take him by auto as he has that fear. But after reaching there, we came to know that the hospital is closed due to some holiday. So the next day, I directly went to the head of the hospital and told her that we had come yesterday and the hospital was closed. She got angry and said that in case of such patients, we have to take the patient immediately for a check-up, and the procedure needs to be initiated immediately. So the head of the hospital immediately typed the memos and gave them to concerned people. I always think, why do such incidents happen? Why don't people do what they are supposed to do? It happened in the police station and hospital as well.

The public prosecutor turned hostile. I don't know why. She would disappear from the hearing after twenty minutes, which is entirely wrong. I had to speak in front of the court alone as she was not there.

During the whole process, I had realised that these people only understand power. When you mention their seniors while talking with them, then they feel some pressure. I went to several police stations, and I am infamous at the police station because of multiple Right to Information (RTI) that I had filed. I filed those RTIs for finding more information as the police's one paper never matches with the other paper, they changed my statement, and my NCs have also changed.

I have been able to master all the steps required for filing of RTI. My children gave me the necessary spirit to be able to do this. I always had the spirit, because of which I could stay in such a situation for so many years. What I am saying is, I tolerated such a man (*asha mansla sahan kela*); it was because I had that spirit.

I also read about the law and got all information on what are my rights, what compensation me and my children will get. I also observed that advocates work very superficially; they don't study the case details to the extent they should. I think if I am in that role, I will study everything about the case in detail. I don't know, maybe because they see such cases every day. Actually, the laws are so good, but nothing happens without proper implementation, and it is not only about my case, but it is the same with everyone's case.

During court hearings, I met many other women who were fighting for domestic violence. There is one friend of mine whose 498A (Section under the Indian Penal Code that criminalises marital violence) has been going on since 1998. She says, "My children got married, my husband remarried, he has kids, and they are also married now."

Coming to my case, I know that the rape law has changed, but my case is of marital rape. I think society has still not accepted that even a woman is an independent individual, and she has a right to say no even if it is a legal marriage. She has first right over her body, and if she does not feel like engaging in a certain sexual act, then it should be respected. If the husband wishes to indulge in the act, then to turn her 'no' into 'yes', he should make some effort. He should take care of her mood, looking after her needs, and instead of opting to violence, he should try to convince her, "I want it, and you can give it to me," not threatening her by saying, "I can get it outside as well."

I will surely say about 498A that with how statements are written, how the police machinery works, and how the court interferes in it, the results of 498A are bound to be bad, and the woman will be blamed for it. The statement which we give, where women say what happened to them, is presented in the court without a signature. Anyone can change the statement as soon as I leave the room. You don't have to even wait for me to reach home. If I can read and write, then why will I not write it in my handwriting? So the police submit such statements to the court, and the court considers them as final. At least women who are educated can write their statements; they can write in their own words, in their handwriting, and if it is not readable, then it can be typed, These are small things, but they matter a lot. Also, there is an obsession for settlement (*settlement cha bhoot itka prachand ahe*), and the court wants to settle the matter one way or another. I have seen that judges put immense pressure on the woman for settlement (*Dokhyavar havi hotat*). I used to strongly tell my mind that I didn't want to do a settlement, but at one point, I felt I was ready for settlement.

There is so much pressure to just finish it, but still, it does not end. The terms of the settlement are also set by the husband, so they are his conditions only. This means we (women) nowhere feel that it is a win-win position. It is not like I lost to some extent, and you also lose to some extent. I lost entirely, I am completely collapsed, and you are the way you were. I have thought that I should write about the preparation that a woman needs to have before she enters the court.

And many women do not have any proof; they ask me, "From where did you bring this?" So even when I explain to them the process, they just keep on looking at me. Sometimes I feel that I collected so many documents, but what happened to them? They are just waste papers (*raddi*) as the order which I was expecting did not come through. They did not mention "rape" while commenting on sexual cruelty; they just left that at one point. Why? I expected them to say that this has happened to me as I mentioned in my complaint to the police. But during my husband's cross-examination, when they asked me, I told them, "Yes, I have spoken about it to Dr B." But in my entire cross-examination, which lasted for four days, the court at no point asked me, "Did it happen forcefully with you?"

I was waiting for them to ask me. Like I had heard stories about the difficult questions that are asked to women (who are raped). The defence lawyers make women cry. I was waiting for that moment, where I could tell that it was like this and not like that. I had completely prepared for that. I used to keep thinking that they might ask me the exact position – where he was and where I was, where my daughter was, where my son was. I had thought a lot and rehearsed in my mind about how I will narrate, but they did not ask anything about it. So the final order mentions physical and mental cruelty but no mention of sexual cruelty. My daughter used to ask why we were destined to have this type of father, and she said to me, "Your youth is wasted because of him." She feels that I could have had a good life and I could have enjoyed my life. Sometimes she messages me, saying, "It was a good decision that we left him. Otherwise, I would have gotten stuck in those four walls." She is 21 years old now.

My son initially had hit a low, but now he is all right. He is a champion in karate and football. It had affected him quite a lot. I used to think, "How am I going to bring him out of this phase?" I used to feel very guilty, that I was responsible for his condition. He used to get very scared, and he would sit in a corner of the house and cry a lot. Even on TV, if there was a mention of the word *baba*, he would immediately curl himself, then we immediately shut down the television or change the topic. There was one counsellor who said to let him face this on TV and talk to him differently. He feels that if you are not strong, you should show him through your actions that you are strong. I did that. Once I came from high court and was very frustrated. I was telling it to my daughter, so he came and held my hand and said, "I feel you are strong now." At that time, I felt like I got a prize! So I thought nothing good happened with me in court, but my son now feels that his mother has become strong.

9 Way forward

The experiences of survivors and their families with the community and the CJS reflect the deep impact it has had on their lives. Of all the women who had come to the hospital, contact could be established with only 25% of them. Of the 66 who participated in the study, 30 required support and intervention, but they had never contacted the counsellor or expressed the need in any earlier follow-up call. What this clearly shows is that there is an urgent need for all three institutions – the police, the hospital, and the court – to establish crisis intervention/counselling departments to provide support to every rape survivor.

These services should include access to resources to help survivors navigate the various systems and prevent re-traumatisation or secondary victimisation. The health needs of survivors are not limited to immediate health consequences post-incident. The narratives in this book show how there are long-term health consequences which survivors have to deal with; this includes adjustments and interactions with the larger social environment within their communities and with various institutions. The narratives also highlight that these needs are not limited to the survivor but extend to the family, who often have to live within communities that are hostile and loaded with myths and misinformation about rape. It is evident that much more needs to be done to help survivors and their families to overcome the trauma that they experience every day. Justice in these cases, therefore, does not come from merely punishing the abuser but ensuring that the survivor is able to regain a life of dignity.

Raising awareness about rights and procedures in the aftermath of rape – from the time the rape is recorded and until the court outcome – will make the journey of survivors and their path towards justice more bearable. Lending support to survivors will also enable them to better prepare and deal with the CJS and help them mitigate the insensitive and callous response of duty bearers, which is often seen in cases related to rape and violence against women. The socio-economic consequences of reporting rape also

DOI: 10.4324/9781003281887-10

need greater attention. This includes ensuring access to compensation, support in accessing other welfare schemes, hostels for children, skill building/ vocational training, and services for persons with disabilities. These needs must also be prioritised along with pursuing the case in court.

Taking note of the fact that only 66 of 728 women who reported a case of rape against them at the hospital could be contacted, we need to recognise that all survivors may not wish to seek justice through the CJS. And while these survivors may not wish to pursue a criminal case, they do require support services, such as psychosocial support, healthcare, rehabilitation, and welfare services, to heal from the abuse. It is, therefore, essential for support and welfare services need to be delinked from the police and CJS so that these services are made accessible for all survivors of sexual violence.

Index

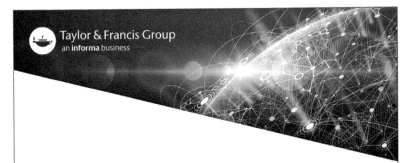

For Product Safety Concerns and Information please contact our EU
representative GPSR@taylorandfrancis.com Taylor & Francis Verlag GmbH,
Kaufingerstraße 24, 80331 München, Germany

Batch number: 08153772

Printed by Printforce, the Netherlands